Healing Fibromyalgia

Why everything hurts and how to feel well again

*Including Dr E's Six-Week
Nearly Natural Cure*

DAVID EDELBERG, MD

WITH HEIDI HOUGH

Healing Fibromyalgia: Why everything hurts and how to feel well again
© 2011 by WholeHealth Chicago

For information on special discounts for bulk purchases, please contact WholeHealth Chicago at 773-296-6700.

Library of Congress Control Number:
ISBN:

Sign up for Dr Edelberg's thought-provoking weekly Health Tips at WholeHealthChicago.com

CONTENTS

1
INTRODUCTION

Fibromyalgia is real. The pain you awaken with is not "in your head." You're not even remotely a hypochondriac. If anyone — any doctor, chiropractor, physical therapist, well-meaning friend, relative, or loved one — ever tries to convince you otherwise, tune them out.

They are wrong.

Likewise, if anyone ever tells you fibro is incurable and you'll just have to learn to live with it, understand they're seriously misinformed.

If you're worried that fibro will develop into something else, like arthritis or a nasty autoimmune disease, let me reassure you right now. Fibro is fibro. Ultimately, when you're very old, you will die (let me be the first to break this terrible news to you), but it won't be from fibromyalgia. The word has never appeared as the cause of death on anybody's death certificate, ever, and never will.

You may have read that many doctors don't believe fibro exists. To my perpetual annoyance, many doctors do feel this way, but fortunately the climate is changing. You can speed the process along by swinging your satchel into your disbelieving doctor's head while shouting, "Learn something about fibromyalgia, you dunderhead!"

Or, if you want to boost the learning curve in a nicer way, at the very end of this book I've included a gift: the Physician's Guide to Fibromyalgia. Just print it out and hand it to your doctor (there's also a printable PDF version at our website, wholehealthchicago.com). If she's forgiven you for the satchel episode, she'll likely find it illuminating (they don't teach this stuff in med school). It's essentially the lecture I've delivered to physicians around the country, and your doctor can e-mail me if he or she has any questions.

It's my hope that with this book and the physician's guide in hand, you and your doctor will become an educated team in treating your fibro.

You may even be able to fix your fibromyalgia on your own, without doctors and without drugs. This book will tell you how.

If you've heard that science doesn't understand fibromyalgia, to this I'd answer, "We may not yet completely grasp everything about it, but we're very close." Certainly by the time you've finished this book, you'll know more about it than most physicians.

As my interest in fibromyalgia grew, the question I kept asking myself was simple: Why are the vast majority of sufferers women? Although men do get fibro, their numbers are miniscule by comparison (less than 5% of people with fibro are male). I needed to know why this gender inequality occurred, and when I figured it out I wasn't at all happy.

Just to give you some advance warning, the original title of this book was to have been *Women Under Siege*. With women facing stress on virtually every front, my thesis is that fibromyalgia has a lot to say about the larger status of women in society.

Be assured I'm not blaming you for your fibromyalgia. If you have it, I ask that you look at your whole self — the mind and body totality that makes you *you* — as being under protective siege, your body trying desperately to guard itself from the assault of multiple sources of stress.

Envision your muscles tightening up and creating a protective suit of armor. That's fibro in a nutshell. It's not a disease. Your muscles aren't sick or inflamed, but they're definitely tired of being locked up like this, trying to protect you and making you utterly exhausted in the process. Ironically, if your muscles could talk, they'd probably say, "Look, lady, we're just doing our job. We got this message from you that we're under serious stress. This tightening-up is what muscles do."

"Wait," you think. "Am I hearing this right? Is he saying that the 12 million American women with fibromyalgia are so stressed that they're engaged in a 24/7 painful muscle lock-up of self protection and self preservation?"

That's exactly what I'm saying.

The statistics prove it: more American women have fibromyalgia than diabetes. What this also means is that some 200 million women around the world are so stressed they're wearing this same painful, locked-up muscle armor. French women. Nigerian women. Vietnamese. Iranian.

200 million women under siege.

All this fibromyalgia, this epidemic. Isn't there a message here? Does this say something about the status of women here on planet Earth? I'm glad you asked and yes, we'll get there.

But in the meantime, let's get rid of your painful fibromyalgia forever.

David Edelberg, MD

2

HOW I BECAME INTERESTED IN FIBROMYALGIA

Fibromyalgia entered my life as the result of a mid-life career change, a decision to exit the world of primary care practice to start a new venture: Opening one of the first integrative medical centers in Chicago.

Combining conventional with alternative medicine was a fairly new concept back then.

Don't get me wrong – I cared deeply about the patients in my internal medicine practice. But I'd grown increasingly disenchanted with my work as a doctor, writing a seemingly endless and not particularly effective stream of prescriptions primarily to relieve symptoms and control diseases brought on by unhealthy living. Nothing I did seemed to be making much difference in anyone's life. Health care felt like the "whack-a-mole" carnival game. Just as soon as we got a patient's blood pressure under control it seemed his cholesterol shot up, so I'd add a new drug for that, but soon my patient was diabetic or seeing a cardiologist for chest pain. Fat people were getting fatter and the tired, more tired.

Yet one group of people I was caring for seemed, provocatively, to be healthier than the rest. These were patients who were using me not as their chief health professional, but rather as one of a group of healers that included nutritionists, chiropractors, acupuncturists, and massage therapists. These patients might need me in a pinch ("Could you sign this form for me?") or to prescribe the infrequently required antibiotic, but generally they took very good care of themselves and required little involvement with conventional doctors.

In medical school, students are taught (subtly or not) that all alternative medicine is pretty much fake. If patients report good results, you're taught that it's either psychological (the placebo effect) or that they would have gotten well anyway. For years, acupuncture was referred to as "quackupuncture" and as for chiropractors, they endured a witch-hunt mentality for years that today is difficult to grasp.

But here I was, seeing the results of alternative medicine — real healing — in my thriving, healthy patients, and I knew I had to learn more about it. I began by asking patients for the names of their practitioners and then calling and asking if I could visit their offices and learn something about what they did. Their responses ranged from enthusiastic to suspicious, but overall our meetings went well, especially when I began referring my patients to them. More often than not, mine was the first inquiry these so-called alternative healers had ever received from a physician.

Even as I was exploring how alternative medicine could be combined with the traditional Western medicine I'd been trained in, a Time Magazine cover article described the medical center of the 21st century as one that would blend conventional and alternative approaches. That's when I decided to quit my job and open Chicago's first such center. Now called integrative medicine, back then we used the word "holistic."

The Chicago Holistic Center (now WholeHealth Chicago)

was busy from day one and has remained so ever since. In a couple of years, we'll have been working together as a group, with me as the MD, for 20 years.

Understand that 20 years ago I knew virtually nothing about alternative medicine. To learn, I attended meetings of the American Holistic Medicine Association, a tiny group (membership about 500, out of 800,000 physicians) of like-minded physicians. I really enjoyed these gatherings. You couldn't help but have fun at a medical meeting where doctors with their grey hair tied back in ponytails wore T-shirts reading "Hugs Heal."

I tried everything, like a kid at a carnival — acupuncture, different kinds of massage, chiropractic adjustments, and chakra balancing. This beat AMA meetings hands-down! And there, for the first time, I heard talks by the early heavy hitters in holistic medicine — Deepak Chopra, Bernie Siegel, Larry Dossey, Andrew Weil, Christiane Northrup, and Carolyn Myss.

I read extensively about the history of healing and tried every so-called alternative medical procedure I could find. This approach, I quickly saw, presented an entirely new toolbox with which to treat my patients. In conventional medicine, drugs take center stage. With integrative medicine, I could use the best of both worlds. I was excited then, and many years later I still am.

Listening to our bodies

At the heart of holistic medicine is the concept of treating the whole person — mind and body — rather than focusing on a symptom or an abnormal physical finding (like high blood pressure) or lab test (like high cholesterol). Today I work with my patients to explore what a particular symptom is trying to convey. *Why* the headaches, *why* the fatigue? When patients understand the message and act on it, more often than not the symptom simply goes away (fibro's more complicated, but stay with me here).

The price of ignoring the message? Generally the symptom gets worse. It's sort of like your house being on fire and a neighbor calling frantically to let you know so you can escape. But you don't want to be bothered, so you let your phone keep ringing.

Let's say, for example, you get a headache every day in the late afternoon and you're tired of it and go to your doctor. Conventional physicians would probably begin by recommending a headache medicine—Tylenol, ibuprofen, or the like. When that doesn't work and you're back at your doc's office, she might order some blood tests, maybe an MRI of your brain, or refer you to a headache specialist for more tests. Weeks and months later, you're relieved that all your tests are normal and you don't have a brain tumor, but your head still hurts every afternoon.

In holistic medicine, the main question is always, "Let's talk about your life." I would ask you to tell me about a "headache day." And after some conversation, it emerges that your headaches occur most often when you skip lunch or replace lunch with a Twinkie and diet cola. Or, when you realize you don't have headaches on weekends, that it's too much time sitting in one position in front of a computer screen. Or on days when your boss is being really nasty or your partner has been drinking a lot and you tense up at the thought of going to work or going home in the evening.

How your biography influences your biology

As I write this now, I'm astonished how totally new this

concept of "biography as biology" was to me back then. Understand, I'd been a primary care doctor for more than 15 years and not once had I been advised to consider a patient's life story, decade by decade. I remember thinking at the time, "Why was I not taught this in medical school?"

I'd first come across this biography-biology concept during a lecture by psychologist and medical intuitive Carolyn Myss, PhD, at one of those American Holistic Medical Association meetings. Later, I would read her books including the impressive *Why People Don't Heal*. In it she explores the common problem of people with chronic symptoms and negative test results, delving into how such symptoms develop and what might be done to help.

The heart of the matter, I soon came to realize, was (and continues to be) an essential flaw in the education of virtually all doctors – namely, an almost willful ignorance of the patient's full life story. This failure to recognize how a person's biography might influence her biology can place a real barrier between an ill patient and her doctor's efforts to help.

And sadly, two decades later, when doctors-in-training sit in with me to hear a "biographical patient interview" (as opposed to the conventional symptom-based one), they're as taken aback as I was long ago by the revelations they hear as my patient reveals her life story.

On to fibromyalgia

So in 1993 or thereabouts, the Chicago Holistic Center has opened. There's me, as the MD, surrounded by a bevy of chiropractors, acupuncturists, homeopaths, bodyworkers, and herbalists, and our schedules are filling up. I've been studiously reframing my interviewing techniques according to ideas from holistic physicians I'd met at the meetings.

No longer will my new-patient interview begin with the standard med-school phrase "When did you first experience symptoms?" Instead I would say "Let's talk about your life," "Tell me when you last felt well," and "Let's go into real detail about the transitional time when you went from feeling just fine, to feeling how you are now. I need to know what was going on during the weeks or months before your symptoms first appeared."

As Dr. Carolyn Myss said in one of her talks, "Most people will look surprised at this line of questioning and say 'No one's ever asked me that before.' Also, when they recall when they did feel fine, expect tears as they remember how little they appreciated good health. But during these minutes, you'll learn a lot about what's going on."

Just a few weeks after we opened, I began to notice I was hearing variations of the same life story. These were women, somewhere between 20 and 60, coming in for help with longstanding symptoms. They'd all been told by other doctors, "We can't find anything wrong with you. Your tests are normal."

If there was one underlying symptom, it was fatigue. Many also described chronic headaches and muscle aching and used phrases like "I feel old!"

At the time, there had been a lot of articles about chronic fatigue syndrome, and no one (doctors or patients) understood anything about it. The very word fibromyalgia was new and not yet connected with chronic fatigue. Articles in medical journals were scanty. It took until 1987 for the AMA to classify fibromyalgia as a legitimate condition and it wasn't until 1990 that the American

Rheumatologic Association provided criteria to teach physicians how to diagnose it.

Remember, this is well before the internet, and almost 20 years before TV ads for FDA-approved drugs for fibromyalgia began to appear and ramp up everybody's learning curve about fibro.

But even when articles on fibro began to appear in medical journals, the vast majority of physicians remained highly skeptical about its existence. Fibromyalgia broke all the rules about disease they'd learned in medical school. There were no positive test results for it, no characteristic x-ray findings — even biopsies of muscle were normal.

To an old-school physician, no positive test results means that no disease is present in the patient. No disease means there's no such thing as fibromyalgia, and that, as they say, is that.

Just a couple of miles away from our fledgling Chicago Holistic Center was a huge major university hospital complex. Deep within the Department of Rheumatology, the rheumatologists agreed there was no such animal as fibromyalgia and that all these women who had widespread muscle aching, fatigue, and depression simply needed a good psychiatrist.

The psychiatrists didn't know what to do either. The women with all these unverifiable symptoms certainly weren't neurotic, and if their pain was real (there was no reason to think otherwise), then they must have been depressed because they felt crummy all the time. So the psychiatrists sent these women back to the rheumatologists, who then returned them to the primary care physicians who'd sent them to the huge medical center in the first place.

Diagnosis: No disease found.

And so, tired and achy, some of the women with what we now know is fibro picked up copies of that Time Magazine (or any of dozens of other magazines writing about alternative medicine) and said to their friends, their partners, or even their physicians, "I think I'm going to give it a try."

One after another, women started making appointments with us. And I, using my shiny new biographically oriented interviewing techniques, listened as the stories of their lives—childhood events, teenage years, marriage, children, and beyond—were described in vivid detail.

And as my patients' lives unfolded before me, I began to realize they described epic stories of fibromyalgia.

Each new patient was like a novel, each was unique in her individual biography, but so many of the stories had striking parallels: My father was a rage-alcoholic...mom was depressed...my migraines began when I was in my teens along with my PMS...they put me on Prozac in college after I was sexually assaulted...I wear a night guard for my TMJ...my muscle pain got worse when dad got cancer and I was the only one to take care of him.

These descriptions—a perfect storm of women under enormous stress—is how I became interested in fibromyalgia. And I have my patients to thank for leading me to the place where I finally understood what was going on.

3

NICOLE'S STORY AND THE EPIC TALE OF FIBRO EXPLAINED

In the "How Can We Help?" section of our WholeHealth Chicago Patient Questionnaire, Nicole had written "I'm in constant pain as long as I can remember and I'm so tired I can't even think straight."

Even as I welcomed her to our center, I noticed how slowly she moved, her muscles stiff. The deeply etched lines around her eyes revealed a daily struggle with constant pain. And yet she was young, not yet 35.

Patient Stories: Nicole

Before I could ask her anything, Nicole initiated the conversation. "I don't mean to be rude, but you're my sixth doctor and if you want to tell me this is all in my head or that I'm depressed, I'll save you the time and me the money and I'll leave. I read an article about fibromyalgia and I think that's what I have. The first four doctors told me my tests were normal and to take it easy. The fifth said I was depressed and to take an antidepressant. Of course I'm depressed. I'm in pain every single day."

I leaned back in my chair. "OK, let's take it slowly, Nicole. Pretend your life is on videotape. Press the rewind button and go back to a time when you felt just fine. No pain, energy good, no health issues—nothing. A time when you took good health for granted,

---

like people who feel fine usually do."

Nicole was silent for almost a full minute as her eyes filled with tears. "I'm sorry, doctor—I'll get control in a minute." I handed her a tissue and she sighed slowly. "It's just that I'm just realizing how long I've felt this way. How many days I've woken up in pain. How many...years, actually."

"OK, so we're back in time now. Pain-free. When is this? Where are you in your life?"

"Oh, you won't have time for this. It's really too long..."

"No—it's fine. Just tell me when."

"I think maybe just before the time my mother was dying and my life fell apart. It was terrible. She had cancer, dad had died the year before, and there was only me to take care of mom. Frank, my husband, had just lost his job and we were living on my income and his unemployment checks. Frank Jr was five or maybe six and sick all the time with his tonsils. I was *always* in a doctor's office with someone and we came this close (she held up two fingers) to losing our home."

"And you started hurting?"

"It seemed like nothing at first—like the aching when you get the flu. Frank would rub my neck and back and I'd feel OK, but in the morning I'd wake up and think: Why am I still *so tired*? Just walking to the bathroom made me feel like I was 90, like I was coming apart. This went on for weeks and I thought, 'I'm only 33. What if I live the next 40 years feeling like this?'

Then my mother passed away. Frank Jr outgrew his tonsil problems—he's 13 now. And my husband finally got a job, but our marriage didn't survive. He was drinking and getting abusive. He started reminding me of my father and I wasn't going that route again. I don't even want to tell you about my childhood."

"But it does sound like your life regained some semblance of order."

Nicole smiled. "I really didn't do too badly for a single mom, and I finally got to use my business degree. Now I make a decent living, though I still struggle through every single day, especially mid-afternoon, when I feel like a truck hit me. My son is my best friend and doing very well in school, but I can barely do the things for him I know he needs—like homework and watching sports. I'm sure he's really tired of hearing me complain about how much I hurt."

"And how's the job?"

She laughed for the first time since we'd met. "Stress follows me everywhere. I went into PR and you'd never believe the stress. My supervisor is sick all the time from the stress she says the VP gives her. And the clients! It's always more, more, more. You don't need to hear all about this. Trust me, every day is a battle and I don't do anything outside of work except what Frank Jr needs."

We discussed the details of her childhood and adolescence with her angry alcoholic father, the fibro-triggering stress of her mother's illness and death, financial pressure, and her husband's drinking and the subsequent divorce. Then we went over the other symptoms that had started cropping up through the years. Chronic sinus congestion, irritable bowel, PMS, poor concentration, all low-serotonin disorders.

Despite tentatively starting a new and promising relationship with Mark, a single dad in the neighborhood, Nicole told me she had no interest in sex. "I know he's going to leave me. I feel fried and I hurt all the time and I'm no fun to be around." And then she paused. "I can't believe my body is such a wreck. And I can't imagine what it's like to feel well."

I looked over all the records Nicole had brought with her. It came as no surprise that all her tests were normal. Then, during the physical exam, 18 of the 18 hallmark fibromyalgia tender points were so painful to light pressure that minutes after the exam she was still hurting. "Is it hopeless?" she asked. "Am I really crazy?"

Reassuring her that not only was she perfectly sane, but that all her symptoms were quite genuine, I agreed that the only reason she could be called depressed was her completely rational response to feeling awful day after day with no light at the end of the tunnel.

Fibro is your low-serotonin body's response to chronic stress

Nicole and I spent some time discussing the human body's physical response to chronic stress. Initiated in the brain, which sends signals to the adrenal glands (which in turn release several hormones that produce our fight-or-flight response), I told Nicole this bodily response was meant to be a brief on-off reaction lasting just a few minutes, the amount of time it takes to escape a mugger or veer your car away from a potential accident. If you picture this stress response as a switch, it's certainly not meant to remain in the "on" position day in and day out.

"Like it is with me?"

"Exactly. And what happens next is that your body sends you symptoms of distress. These signals mean there's trouble somewhere, and your irritable bowel, PMS, and lack of concentration are all low-serotonin symptoms of something called the fibromyalgia spectrum. Symptoms don't necessarily mean you have a disease. They're a signal that something needs attention."

"But what if you try to get help with the signals, like I did, and you don't get any help?"

"Well, your body starts undergoing changes. And those changes, like the PMS or the brain fog or the constant pain and tenderness of your muscles, and any of a dozen other symptoms..."

"...are fibro?"

"You got it. Fibromyalgia means 'muscle pain' in Greek. For a lot of doctors, fibro doesn't fulfill what we learned in medical school about the definition of disease. It's not an autoimmune disorder. It's not an infection. It's not contagious. No one ever dies of it. The blood tests, x-rays—even biopsies that we use to diagnose other diseases—are all normal. But obviously, it's something. You feel terrible! And, there are 12 million women like you here in the US."

Nicole's treatment plan

We spent the rest of the visit going over a treatment plan that would slowly but surely move her body out of constant stress mode. I asked three things of Nicole before we met again:

- **First, I wanted her to carefully review her life and examine all sources of stress.** Maybe it would be reconsidering her job and switching to a less stressful firm. Some companies seem to pride themselves on creating stress as a way of life for their employees. She should practice the word "no" (pronounced "no") when others piled demands on her. And she was to start some pleasurable activities. A morning walk. Time spent reading. Going somewhere with her son. Some very limited gentle exercise.

- **Second, I wanted her to start taking a combination of nutritional supplements.** Nicole was adamant about not taking pharmaceuticals as a first step, having experienced awful side effects from most every drug she'd ever taken. We agreed she'd start on the supplement regimen and see if she got some relief, though I asked her to keep an open mind about taking tiny doses of fibro drugs if this path didn't pan out. I warned her in advance that the supplements would seem like a lot of pills to swallow, but these weren't forever. My goal was twofold. We wanted her symptoms relieved: Better sleep, less pain, more energy, better mood, no PMS. But we also wanted to start repairing some of the damage to her body that the years of chronic stress had inflicted.

- **Third, I wanted her to begin sessions with a myofascial release massage therapist** (page 254) to start the process of releasing her locked-up muscles. I told her how important it was to know the sensation of feeling good again—of being pain-free—even if at first it was only temporary. She needed this sense of hope, a taste of the possibilities of wellness that lay ahead. To understand how her muscles had "remembered" the repeated stressful assaults of her raging alcoholic father so long ago, I also asked her to read Memories in Your Muscles (page 57).

For me to tell you that Nicole's fibro was cured in three weeks would not only be deceptive, but just plain silly. If only life worked such miracles! But after just five weeks following the plan laid out in the Nearly Natural Fibro Cure (page 103), Nicole told me she was undeniably aware of changes going on in her body. And these were changes for the better.

As months passed and I saw less of Nicole, I learned from other therapists in our office what was happening. She'd left her job and found a position for a little less money, but with a fraction of the pressure, a shorter commute, and one day a week working from home. Nicole herself had used the Nearly Natural Cure to reframe her life, focusing on eating nutritionally powerful foods and exercising routinely.

She'd also been journaling and one day told me she now recognized how extreme the stress had been, growing up with her father. "I started to understand what you meant about muscles remembering, and also I forgave myself for feeling so awful all these years," she told me.

Nicole was finding yoga classes incredibly helpful, both for body and mind, and she said the guided imagery "was like a vacation." During brief follow-up visits with me for a cold or Pap smear, we trimmed her supplement list until she was down to some basic vitamins and a healthy bone supplement.

And Nicole's fibro began drifting to the back burner of her life.

One year later, this is what she told me:

"It's not gone, like gone-gone, but I rarely have any muscle pain anymore. And my irritable bowel is completely gone and the PMS just about. My energy has zoomed up—enough to have a standing Sunday date with Mark and his son, me, and Frank Jr.

"But I have to tell you the muscles in my neck are like radar. If they start tensing up, I scan the horizon. 'OK,' I ask myself, 'what's going on in my life?' I realized months ago that there will always be stuff happening to stress me out. That's life. But I can choose to not give in to it. I made some changes to step away from that stress and so far it's working."

And then she thanked me and gave me a hug. I knew Nicole would be OK.

Fibromyalgia explained

Fibro affects more than 12 million people, the vast majority of them women.

And though there's a Fibromyalgia Awareness Month each year, many sufferers who have lived with widespread muscle pain for decades are already plenty "aware" of their fibro. Then there are others, like the 71-year-old woman I saw recently whose fibro began when she was about 25. After several doctors told her "it was all in her head," she had accepted this (hogwash) as truth.

A half century of constant daily pain is so unimaginable that simply for her we should all learn more about fibro and share the information. You get an idea of the frustration fibro patients feel by looking at websites like Fighting Fatigue, the National Fibromyalgia Association, and Focus on Fibromyalgia Inc (better known by its web address: fibromyalgiasucks.org and, yes, t-shirts are available).

Doctors who "care for" people with undiagnosed fibro are almost always no help whatsoever

Patient surveys confirm that the typical woman with fibromyalgia sees five physicians before she actually learns she has fibro. Until the internet broadened awareness of the condition, most gave up after two or three doctors and accepted pain as their lot in life. For the diligent ones, that fifth doctor probably said something like: "Well, I'm sorry to tell you this. It appears you have fibromyalgia. We don't know much about it. Here's an antidepressant. Since it's not a disease, there's really not much we can do about it. Go exercise—that's supposed to help."

But because deep fatigue accompanies fibro pain, when the person with fibro tries to follow her doctor's recommendation to exercise she finds she can barely manage a fraction of what she handled with ease just a few years earlier.

In fact, Fibromyalgia Awareness Month should be directed at the entire medical profession, including chiropractors. I have some experience in this area. During the past few months, I've been all over the country giving lectures to physicians about fibro, and their overall lack of knowledge is appalling.

Most of the doctors I've met say they "never see fibro" in their practices or at the most have one or two patients, whom they refer to rheumatologists. Many still believe there's "no such condition" and consider it "basically psychiatric," referring their patients to a psychiatrist. These are actual quotes from physicians I've met with and they are wrong, wrong, wrong.

Remember the game "hot potato"?

That's the way most fibromyalgia patients are treated, tossed around from one medical professional to the next. If you've traversed the medical system with fibro, I'm not telling you anything new.

Many rheumatologists also believe fibromyalgia is a

psychiatric disorder. Psychiatrists don't understand fibro at all and wonder why the rheumatologist referred the patient to them. After realizing the patient referred for alleged depression is basically (and reasonably) depressed because of chronic pain, the psychiatrist refers her to a pain management specialist. Pain specialists have told me they regard fibro patients as "needy and time consuming."

Psychiatrists may not be recognizing vast numbers of fibromyalgia patients because this particular specialty, fearing malpractice over "inappropriate behavior," has become phobic about performing physical examinations on their patients. Fibro is painfully (pardon the pun) simple to diagnose. All that's necessary is for the doctor to apply firm pressure to fibromyalgia's 18 classic tender points and watch the patient's startled reaction to the jolt of pain the pressure induces.

What a mess this all is for the woman in chronic daily pain. And believe me if any of these doctors actually had fibro, he'd be in the back seat of his BMW being driven to Mayo Clinic for help this afternoon. What he doesn't know is that Mayo would turn him away—they're already swamped with fibro patients and would tell him that his local doctor should be able to manage the case as effectively as they could. Except of course, he is "the local doctor" and clueless about what's wrong with him.

But doctors are not managing fibro because it doesn't fit with their training

Most physicians simply don't get it when it comes to fibro, and the reason for this is a single glaring deficiency in medical education. As medical students, doctors learn that symptoms without corresponding disease somewhere in the body are not to be taken as seriously as symptoms caused by a specific disease.

Headaches are thus less compelling without a brain tumor to treat. Back pain is of routine interest until disc surgery is in order.

When you tell your doctor about your symptoms ("I have a headache" or "I'm tired"), your physician is trained to look for an underlying disease responsible for your discomfort. He or she orders tests—blood tests, imaging, biopsies—a cornucopia of tests. If the tests show *something*, treatment will be started with the goal of curing you and relieving your symptoms.

If, however, the tests come up normal (as they do with fibro), to the doc's way of thinking his or her responsibilities are basically over. You're reassured your symptoms are harmless and maybe get a prescription for a pill that might relieve (or mask) your symptoms. Intellectually, your physician is off the hook. Occasionally you might be referred to another physician who orders a different battery of tests, but generally doctors become less and less interested in you because to their way of thinking, there's nothing wrong with you...nothing to "cure."

I've had patients who told me that other doctors asked "Aren't you pleased to learn nothing serious is going on? You should be relieved we can't find anything wrong with you. All your tests are normal."

But you're not feeling in any way normal. If you have undiagnosed fibromyalgia, you're thinking, "All this pain, this fatigue—it can't be normal." If you know you have fibro and you're told, "There's nothing we can do," then life looks very bleak indeed.

But please believe me: There is hope for people with fibro and this book contains the recipe for getting better. But before we get there, let's review a few facts about fibro.

Stress, low-serotonin disorders, the fibromyalgia spectrum, and fibro pain

To understand fibro pain, you need to understand serotonin, the brain chemical (neurotransmitter) that acts as your buffer against stress. Women have lower levels of serotonin than men, and as a consequence women are more vulnerable to stress of any kind. Some women have it even worse, coming from families at the very low end of the serotonin curve. These families have an even higher rate of low-serotonin disorders, including fibromyalgia.

Women whose low serotonin makes them particularly susceptible to stress are sensitive to everything. They feel potentially painful stimulus (like an inflated blood pressure cuff) more strongly than others and are unusually sensitive to certain foods, chemicals, and drug side effects. They're also extremely aware of changes in their body, *feel* their hormone fluctuations, *know* when a food is wrong for them, and *sense* negative energy from an indifferent or impatient physician. Interestingly, low-serotonin women are often creative and highly intuitive, frequently needing to explain what's obvious (to them) to otherwise clueless men.

Men, of course, are not immune to low-serotonin disorders, but statistically women far outnumber them.

It's also worth noting that all the low-serotonin disorders were once thought to be all psychological in nature. The list included depression, anxiety, panic attacks, obsessive thinking, compulsive behaviors, social anxiety, post-traumatic stress disorder, anger issues (common in men), and self-medication tendencies using food (especially carbs), and alcohol and other drugs.

. Why are the antidepressant herb St. John's wort and the SSRI family of antidepressants (Prozac, Zoloft, Lexapro, et al) effective against all these disorders? Because they boost serotonin levels in the brain.

How low serotonin leads to fibromyalgia spectrum disorders and fibro pain

Researchers in fibromyalgia began seeing so many conditions associated with it they began using the medical term "co-morbidities." I myself dislike anything using the word "morbid" and thus prefer "fibromyalgia spectrum disorders." These include all the psychological mood disorders listed above *plus* all the manifestations of being an extremely sensitive person (the reactions to food, drugs, and chemicals that make up multiple chemical sensitivity syndrome) *plus* manifestations of an unchecked fight-or-flight response, like tension/migraine headaches, jaw clenching/TMJ, irritable bowel syndrome, PMS, and adrenal/thyroid/ovarian fatigue.

The physical manifestations of low-serotonin, fibromyalgia spectrum disorders occur when your body itself experiences unchecked stress. Everyone—male or female, fibro or not— has the potential to feel these fight-or-flight symptoms. It's just that low-serotonin women feel them more than anyone else. As I explained to Nicole, your fight-or-flight response is meant to be a quick on-off system that gets you out of trouble. It's supposed to shoot you full of adrenalin so you can move with lightning speed to avoid an oncoming car, for example. But for stressed-out, low-serotonin women, it's like the fight-or-flight "on" button is pressed down and held there, putting their stress response systems into constant overdrive. After a time, the body simply can't cope.

Most people first notice the physical manifestations of stress as constant tension in the muscles of their neck and upper back. These muscles fan out over the top of the head (producing tension headaches), jaw (jaw-clenching TMJ), and face (felt as a pressure sensation, often incorrectly diagnosed as sinus headache). Migraines are involved here, too, when arteries deep in the brain start contracting in response to stress messages.

If you observe women in a workplace, someone's always reaching behind to massage a knot in her shoulder or tilting her head back to dig in and loosen her neck muscles. When muscles start tightening up over your entire body, you're entering fibro pain territory.

The extremely painful tender points of fibro are small areas where muscles attach to bone. Once tender points are activated, it becomes painful to sit for long periods, find a comfortable position for sleep, or even fall asleep at all. A diagnosis of fibromyalgia depends on the existence of these tender points, and doctors who understand fibro and apply about ten pounds of fingertip pressure to them will get a response like "Gee, doc, that REALLY HURTS!"

Easing fibro pain

To be fair, doctors face a real challenge when treating fibro.

- **First, fibro patients are extremely chemically sensitive,** probably related to their low levels of stress-buffering serotonin. If anyone is going to experience a side effect from medications, it will be a fibro patient. That's why many of my patients begin by taking the supplements listed in the Nearly Natural Cure (page 103).

• **Second, fibro drugs taken at recommended doses actually have more side effects** than most other prescription medicines. I've personally sampled them all on myself, just to anticipate what side effects my patients might experience, and I don't regard myself as particularly chemically sensitive, but all things considered I would have preferred sampling a selection of Cote du Rhone wines. However, as you'll read in Medications for Fibro (page 187), by taking the small doses I recommend you can largely side-step side effects while targeting the unique pain of fibro.

There are three FDA-approved drugs for fibro. Two of them, Savella and Cymbalta, were originally developed as antidepressants, but were later found to have fibro pain-relieving benefits. Physiologically, they do correct the basic underlying issue with fibro—low levels of the brain chemicals serotonin and norepinephrine—and ease pain for about half the women who try them. The other half are stymied by the side-effects of these meds, which include nausea, headaches, palpitations, and sweating, though these can be mitigated by taking the drugs in much smaller doses.

The third FDA-approved med is Lyrica, one of several in a class of anti-epilepsy drugs that some years ago was found to have pain-reducing qualities. Lyrica works for about a third of my patients who try it, the other two-thirds abandoning it due to side effects including dizziness, brain fog, double vision, and weight gain. Again, I prescribe a far lighter dose regimen, presented in the medications chapter.

I also prescribe pain drugs for fibro pain, again in small doses. Many physicians won't even consider giving a woman with fibro a pain medicine, and I believe this is not only heartless but cruel. More about pain and how I recommend you tackle it in Pain Drugs for Fibro (page 227).

Fibro in a nutshell

Here's a fibro diagnosis short list: You've had three or more months of widespread muscle pain and chronic tiredness, 11 of your 18 tender points elicit an "Ow!" response when tested, your tender points have a right-left symmetry, and your tender points are above and below the belt-line.

Each of these low-serotonin symptoms—the pain, exhausttion, and response to tender point pressure—is a physiological response to stress and not a disease. As crazy as it may seem, your body is reacting in the way it's supposed to react, given excessive stress and your insuffic-ient stress buffer. But because your body's response is not a disease, finding a cause for these symptoms flies under the radar of blood tests, x-rays, and other diagnostic tests. In other words, "Your tests are normal."

A few review notes:

- **Fibro is one of the low-serotonin fibromyalgia spectrum disorders,** a group of often disabling conditions that manifest themselves among genetically susceptible people (mainly women) after a period in their lives of unchecked stress.

- **Because of the relationship between serotonin and estrogen,** the severity of any low-serotonin disorder (but especially fibro) parallels your estrogen level. Hence, symptoms worsen during PMS days and pre-menopause, when your estrogen levels are dropping. Most women feel a tad better the week after their periods, when estrogen (and serotonin) levels are rising. Most also feel better in summer than winter because sunshine boosts serotonin levels.

- **Low-serotonin disorders can begin at any age when stress exceeds your stress buffer.** My youngest fibro patient was eight years old. Serotonin disorders like childhood depression and anxiety have reached epidemic proportions. One recent report estimated that 10% of the US population over age 9 is taking serotonin-boosting SSRI antidepressants.

- **From a biographical perspective, fibro usually follows a highly stressful year from hell** in a woman's life. Your fibro-triggering stress might have come from job, family situation, financial situation, injury or serious illness, or simply from living in a stressful world.

- **"Time heals all wounds" ought to apply.** Most stressful life events recede, given enough time. But for fibro patients, they're replaced by the stress of fibro itself with its relentless widespread pain, profound fatigue, unrefreshing sleep, and a medical system ("We can't find anything wrong with you") that doesn't know how or exactly what to treat ("I'm referring you to a ..."). Soon the quest to simply feel normal again becomes life's major source of stress.

Fibro begins with stressors that trigger painful muscle contractions. Now that same pain exacerbates stress, which further increases pain levels. An evil snowball of pain, rolling down a mountain, larger and larger, out of control.

The Fatigue of Fibro
Right up there with pain, the second most common fibro

symptom is a constant sense of profound exhaustion. Disability insurance companies, people who don't have fibro, and (sadly) most doctors can't appreciate the extraordinary degree of this fatigue.

It's not easy for people who don't have fibro to imagine waking up achy all over, feeling as if you'd never really slept, and then staggering through your day before crashing between 2 and 5 pm with even more fatigue. If you actually do have fibro, at this point you've probably tried fortifying yourself with a Starbucks, but what you really want is to crawl into bed. You plan no evening activities and you say "sorry, I can't" to most invitations. Your house is a mess and your significant other is not happy with you being exhausted all the time since your doctor has told you "all your tests are normal."

It's taken scientists about 40 years to figure out where this fatigue comes from. In the 1960s, when fibro itself was barely known, reports of patients who were constantly tired and felt flu-like achiness and poor sleep began to appear in medical journals. All the tests for fatigue were negative for the usual conditions, and some years later the mysterious condition was nicknamed "yuppie flu." Later it would be called chronic fatigue syndrome (CFS).

In an attempt to find a culprit for CFS, researchers pointed to variety of infections, including chronic mononucleosis, herpes, cytomegalovirus, candida (a yeast), and the then newly discovered Lyme disease, but nothing consistently shown to cause CFS. A patient support group named their condition "chronic fatigue immune dysfunction syndrome" (CFIDS) based on the belief that a compromised immune system was the cause, but again, this wasn't supported by research.

Now it's pretty much agreed that fibromyalgia and CFS are one and the same.

Several factors occur simultaneously to induce fibro fatigue

The most significant is how the human body responds to chronic stress. Please don't feel bad if you have to read this next explanation a couple of times. Med students have to memorize all this and don't enjoy it one bit.

As discussed earlier, when you experience a stressful event your body goes into a temporary fight-or-flight response. The full pathway, which operates at blazing speed when needed, looks like this:

- A stress message from your conscious brain sends two signals at lightning-fast speed. The first goes directly to your adrenal glands by way of a set of nerves called the autonomic nervous system, triggering a release of adrenalin, the fight-or-flight hormone. This places your body into temporary overdrive. It's this rush of adrenalin that gives a woman the super-human strength to lift a car off her toddler. The second signal travels to your brain's hypothalamus, which then shoots it over to the brain's pituitary (the master gland), which in turn releases adrenocortical stimulating hormone (ACTH), triggering the release of a second adrenal hormone called cortisol. Cortisol helps you adjust to chronic stress by producing a variety of subtle metabolic changes throughout the body, some of which (like abdominal weight gain) we'd all rather do without.

The full pathway—brain-to-adrenal glands **plus** brain-to-pituitary-to-adrenal glands—is the human stress response.

The second pathway alone is commonly called the HPA axis (hypothalamic-pituitary-adrenal axis).

Your brain-to-adrenal glands pathway is generally pretty resilient, capable of dealing with life's little stressors (dog throwing up on your rug, traffic, bicycle messengers) all day long. But you need to imagine a sign dangling from your HPA axis that reads "WARNING: For emergency use only." That's the way it *should* be. The delicate HPA axis is protected by stress-buffering serotonin. If you're a low-serotonin person and life's stresses (bad boss, financial strain, sick child, too much responsibility) exceed your stress buffer, your HPA axis is activated again and again.

If your stressful life simply won't let up, you exhaust your HPA system.

When you see the phrase "adrenal fatigue" or a natural practitioner says "you've fried your adrenals," this is what's being described. Conventional physicians rarely test patients for adrenal fatigue and generally are unaware of its existence. That's because adrenal fatigue is not a disease, but rather a physiologic response (your overused HPA axis) gone awry.

In addition, with this longer-lasting chronic stress (months on end of real-life stressors, but not the car-lifting type) your pituitary releases a second hormone called TSH (thyroid stimulating hormone) to boost levels of thyroid hormone. TSH is needed to help your metabolism adjust to chronic stress. The thyroid controls the rate of your metabolism— how slow or fast your incredibly complex body will run.

During the initial days and even weeks of stress, you'll have elevated levels of both thyroid and adrenal hormones, the increase being part of your normal stress response. But over time—and during the relentless stress of fibro—the HPA axis, including the thyroid and even sometimes your sex glands (ovaries and testicles, also under pituitary control), begin to become "exhausted" as well.

Thus the primary source of fatigue in fibro is the exhaustion of the HPA axis and thyroid gland, both of which started out trying to protect you but dropped from exhaustion along the way. And this intricate action flies under the radar of conventional doctors testing for fatigue.

Here's how fatigue symptoms present themselves

- **Thyroid fatigue** produces pervasive tiredness, dry skin, dry hair, weight gain, and cold hands and feet. The standard test result for an underfunctioning thyroid is high TSH (thyroid-stimulating hormone). But because TSH comes from your pituitary and it's exhausted too, your TSH is spuriously low. And patients hear, "You can't have an underactive thyroid—your TSH is low."

- **Adrenal fatigue** also brings overwhelming fatigue, along with a mid-afternoon crash of still more exhaustion between 2 and 5 pm. This occurs because you have a one-day supply of hormones in your adrenal glands that need to be restored each night during sleep. They aren't replenished if, like most fibro patients, you're not sleeping well.

- **Ovarian fatigue** leads to irregular periods, worsening PMS, infertility issues, and low or nonexistent sex drive.

In addition to exhaustion of the HPA axis, there are three unrelated sources of fibro fatigue

- **Chronic pain from any source** — whether from fibro, arthritis, or cancer — is itself exhausting.

- **People with fibro sleep very poorly.** Unable to find a comfortable position in bed, you rarely achieve the deep, restorative sleep necessary for normal next-day activities. You awaken exhausted, feeling as though you hadn't slept at all.

- **Eventually the muscles of fibro patients atrophy.** Many who suffer with fibro live a bed-to-chair existence because they're exhausted and in pain. But not moving just makes fatigue worse.

One last word about the long-ago suspected immune dysfunction of fibro-CFS. A well-conducted clinical study at Chicago's DePaul University some years ago did come up with two positive tests among their hundreds of patients. One test showed evidence of adrenal fatigue. The other revealed minimal dysfunction of the immune system, basically the same abnormalities you'd expect if an immune system were experiencing unchecked stress and wasn't functioning efficiently.

In other words, the mono, herpes, candida, et. al., weren't *causing* the fibro-CFS. It was the reverse. The stress of fibro-CFS was impairing the immune system, allowing the emergence of these minor players. For decades, scientists were sidetracked by these microorganisms, believing them to be the "cause" of fibro-CFS, rather than the "result."

Complicated, eh? It's taken decades to figure this out.

Listening for the message your body is conveying

If you have fibro, philosophically understanding what's

occurring in your body is an essential part of treatment. Like Nicole, once you pull back and see the larger fibro picture, you'll realize that all your life you (and likely your mom) have been more susceptible to stress and more sensitive to physical sensations, including pain, than other people.

Identifying the triggering stresses of your fibro is also key, as is developing a plan to lift that stress off your life so you can breathe and start getting well.

As you work with the Nearly Natural Cure (page 103), you'll come to see that fibro is not a disease but rather a defense, and you'll recognize that it will never develop into a disease, but will remain what it is — a stress response from hell — until you acknowledge the message of this pain and take steps to resolve it.

No, I assure you, it's not your fault.

You're a low-serotonin person and your fibro appeared as a response to stressful factors in your life. But there's hope in the step-by-step plan I designed for Nicole and my other patients. You can start that plan today.

Once you free yourself from the pain and you're feeling better, excellent. But if fibro symptoms start to return, don't panic. Rather, regard them as a message that your body is perceiving stress from some source.

With this kind of fibro-flare, it's fine to restart supplements and/or medication, but this time, press the pause button on your life. Seriously reflect on the possible source that's triggering the return of your symptoms. Are you trying to do too much? Have you been neglecting your diet? Is physical activity at a standstill? Are you in a relationship or job that your body *knows* is wrong?

Listen carefully for the message your body is trying to convey and act on it.

If you're just starting the process of healing your fibro, know that when you take steps to resolve these triggers, your muscles will slowly relax, the pain will recede, your body will heal, and many of the meds and supplements I recommend in this book can be tapered off or even discontinued altogether.

In short, you'll get your life back.

4

HOW DO I KNOW IF I HAVE FIBRO?
TAKE THE QUIZ

Even if you've already been diagnosed with fibromyalgia, take the quiz to gain a better understanding of fibro's underpinnings. Because fibro is not a disease per se and offers your doctor no positive test results on which to confirm a diagnosis, 85% of women who have it go undiagnosed, often for years.

A recent survey of physicians revealed 70% of doctors "don't feel competent" to diagnose fibromyalgia...so why not do it yourself?

Part One

1. 95% of people with fibro are female—12 million in the US alone, which means more women have fibro than have diabetes.

   Are you a woman?

   Y - N

2. Fibromyalgia is Greek for "muscle pain." This is an achy sensation in the muscles, usually starting in your neck and upper back.

   Do you carry your stress in your neck, shoulders, and / or upper back?

   Y - N

3. There are certain characteristics of muscle pain that are specific to fibro. The key word is "widespread." Generally, fibro muscle pain starts in your neck, shoulders, and upper back and then spreads, although some women feel it first in their lower back and pelvis. Fibro pain is achy in nature, and though on some days certain areas can hurt more than others, fibro pain is not localized to any one area.

   Is your muscle pain widespread?
   Y - N

4. The second most common symptom of fibro is fatigue, a real sense of tiredness, dragging through the day, having difficulty with work or household chores, crashing at night.

   Do you suffer fatigue?
   Y - N

5. Sleep is a real problem for people with fibro. Patients have difficulty sleeping and often awaken unrefreshed, exhausted and stiff in the morning ("I feel old"), as if they haven't slept at all.

   Do you suffer from unrefreshing sleep and feel stiff and achy when you get up in the morning?
   Y - N

6. People with fibro also have trouble with focus and concentration, called fibro-fog. Simple activities, like balancing a checkbook, become real challenges.

   Do you suffer from poor focus and/or concentration?
   Y - N

7. Stress exacerbates fibro.

   Do your muscles hurt or feel achy most of the time, but

especially when you're stressed?
Y – N

8. Another characteristic of fibro pain is duration, an achiness that's been around at least three months. Again, some days worse than others.

   Have you been in discomfort for three months or longer?
   Y – N

9. Location of muscle pain is also a clue.

   Are you feeling achy in your neck and upper back, on the front of your chest, in your lower back, in both hips, and on the insides of both knees?
   Y – N

10. People with fibro are prone to headaches. These may be tension headaches (a tight band-like headache over the eyes) and/or migraines (throbbing headaches usually on one side of your head, often accompanied by nausea and sensitivity to light).

    Do you suffer frequent tension or migraine headaches?
    Y – N

11. Fibro can mimic other medical conditions, including the early stages of rheumatoid arthritis, lupus, osteoarthritis, hypothyroidism, severe vitamin D deficiency, and the impossible-to-pronounce polymyalgia rheumatica. A few blood tests can quickly rule out these possibilities.

    Has your doctor ruled out other causes of your muscle pain?
    Y – N

12. Fibro can also occur along with any chronic medical condition. Some people being treated for conditions like

rheumatoid arthritis, lupus, or multiple sclerosis seem to reach a plateau with their therapy and get no better, because they have undiagnosed fibro.

If you have a chronic medical condition and are still in pain, has your doctor also considered fibromyalgia?
Y – N

13. Many people being treated for chronic depression or anxiety meet all the criteria for fibro, but have never mentioned their other symptoms to their therapist. Also, many women with chronic pelvic pain who are being evaluated by their gynecologists for fibroids or endometriosis meet all the criteria for fibro.

    Do you have a history of depression, anxiety, or chronic pelvic pain AND do you have widespread muscle achiness that you've never mentioned to your doctor or therapist?
    Y – N

14. Most people with fibro slog through their days doing only what's absolutely necessary (and sometimes not even than much) and not able to do the things that bring them pleasure.

    Do your symptoms interfere with your enjoyment of life?
    Y – N

15. The average fibro patient suffers needlessly for five years (often longer) before learning she has fibro.

    If you sought help for your symptoms, did you hear a variation of "We can't find anything wrong with you – all your tests are normal"?
    Y – N

16. Fibro almost always begins after a period of protracted physical or emotional stress.

    During the months before your symptoms began, were you experiencing an unusual amount of stress in your life?
    Y - N

17. One of the saddest statistics about fibromyalgia is that 25% of patients were psychologically, physically, or sexually abused as children or experienced a sexual assault as young women (date rape).

    Does any of this apply to you?
    Y - N

18. People with fibro are often sensitive to chemicals, feeling nausea or headaches with chemical smells and even perfumes. In addition, they frequently experience side effects from prescription drugs

    Are you chemically sensitive?
    Y - N

19. Fibro patients often have chronic pelvic pain and painful intercourse. They're frequently given such diagnoses as interstitial cystitis, endometriosis, or fibroids. Yet treatment for these conditions fails to bring relief.

    Do you suffer from chronic pelvic pain or painful intercourse?
    Y - N

KEY:
- If you answered yes to questions 3, 4, 5, and 8, you probably have fibromyalgia.
- If you answered no to some of those questions but yes to any of the others, you're at real risk for fibro. Read

Preventing Fibromyalgia (page 289) for ideas on how to avert it.

Part Two

Although chronic muscle pain, exhaustion, poor sleep, and brain fog are the hallmarks of fibro and enough for anyone to endure, a majority of women later diagnosed with fibro first suffered a range of seemingly unrelated low-serotonin symptoms, which I call the fibromyalgia spectrum. For many woman later diagnosed with fibro, these symptoms actually appeared first, years before the widespread muscle pain of their fibro began.

Have you had or do you currently have any of the following low-serotonin symptoms (score 1 point for every yes answer)?

Migraine headaches
Y – N

Irritable bowel syndrome (episodes of bloating, constipation, diarrhea, cramping)
Y – N

Severe PMS (with mood swings)
Y – N

Restless legs at night
Y – N

Cold hands and feet
Y – N

Lightheadedness when standing up quickly
Y – N

Physical symptoms during periods of stress (headaches, stomach aches, TMJ)
Y – N

A tendency to gain weight, but not lose it, despite healthful diet and exercise
Y - N

An injury to your neck or spine from which you feel you've never completely recovered (e.g., a whiplash injury that "never seemed to go away").
Y - N

A worsening of any of these symptoms with weather changes
Y - N

Do you regard yourself as unusually sensitive to the world? This can include being highly intuitive, overreacting to feeling slighted, or being emotionally/physically sensitive to colors, smells, tastes, and sensations—almost as if you've gone through life as a walking "open wound" in a world made of salt?
Y - N

Because the brain needs sunlight to make serotonin, fibro symptoms are often worse in winter, when levels of stress-buffering serotonin drop. This situation is also responsible for the depression of seasonal affective disorder (SAD).

Are your symptoms worse in winter and/or do you experience depression during dark winter months?
Y - N

Because your brain needs carbohydrates to manufacture serotonin, low-serotonin women often crave quickly absorbed "fast carbs" such as bread, chips, pasta, chocolate, and other sweets.

Do you crave fast carbs?
Y - N

Because serotonin levels are linked to estrogen levels, all low-serotonin disorders worsen when estrogen levels drop. These include one week before your period starts (PMS), the six weeks after delivering a baby (post partum depression), and during menopause.

Do any of your low-serotonin symptoms worsen during these times?
Y - N

Have you experienced any of these low-serotonin disorders: depression, anxiety/panic, obsessive thinking, compulsive behavior, social anxiety, phobias, eating disorders, post-partum depression?
Y - N

Low-serotonin disorders run through the women in families. **Did anyone in your biological family — especially the women — have any of the conditions listed just above?**
Y - N

KEY:
If you answered yes to any of these Part 2 questions, it's a clue that you're more sensitive to the world than other women and most men. Recognize this and take good care of yourself, as outlined in Preventing Fibromyalgia (page 289). Understand that if you experience any period of sustained stress in the future, you are at risk for fibromyalgia as well as any of the symptoms listed above.

Next Steps

If your answers lead you to suspect you have fibro or could be at real risk for it, I recommend a twofold path. First, finish reading this book. Then begin the Nearly Natural Cure (page 103). I trust you to know from that single chapter how to proceed.

Fibro Quicksand: Listening to people who say fibro doesn't exist

Tune out anyone—physician, chiropractor, well-meaning friend—who says "there's no such thing as fibromyalgia" or "we don't know anything about it, so there's nothing we can do."

Fibro is real. 12 million-plus women in the US have it, more than have diabetes. But fibro's not a disease like diabetes. Rather, it's a chronic pain syndrome that surfaces in a genetically susceptible person (95% are women and girls), usually after a period of protracted emotional or physical stress.

My patients' fibro has been triggered by the stress of an awful divorce or break-up, an emotionally abusive relationship at work or home, a job from hell, serious financial problems, death of a loved one, physical abuse as a child or adult, serious vehicle accidents, and extensive surgery.

Listening to any uninformed friend or healthcare practitioner tell you fibro doesn't exist has real consequences, since ignoring symptoms allows them to worsen. Although fibro itself doesn't lead to any other serious condition, when fibro pain is allowed to build unchecked for months or years, it becomes harder to treat.

Plus, you need help working through whatever stress has been the catalyst for your fibro.

If you're looking for a knowledgeable and compassionate physician to work with you on the plan in this book, check the helpful web links in Week 1 of the Nearly Natural Cure (page 103).

5

HOW TO CLASSIFY YOUR FIBRO SEVERITY

If you were a fibro patient seeing me for the first time, together we'd try to get a sense of the severity of your symptoms and how they'd affected your life. We'd focus on two specific fibro indicators—pain and fatigue—and our conversation might go something like this, with me starting...

"Think of your very worst fibro pain day and call that a 10. Now go back to when you were completely pain-free. That would be 0. Envision your numbers over the past year. Maybe you were a 10 during the month before you quit your job, a 3 during your Florida vacation this past winter. Now tell me, where have you been, number-wise, during the past two or three months?"

And you'd respond with a fibro pain number, which you can write here _____.

"My goal is to get your pain from there down to a livable 0-1 range. Now let's move on to fatigue. At 10, you're so exhausted can barely operate the remote control on your TV, so tired you're either on medical leave from work or simply can't enter the workforce. But at 0, you have no fatigue whatsoever and you can fully enjoy your day. Where has your fatigue been?

Write your fibro fatigue number here _____.

During every office visit or e-mail exchange with your own physician, I'd like you to evaluate these two symptoms and put a number to them. Of course, be sure to mention other symptoms to your doctor too, like brain fog, insomnia, or medication side effects. Take a look at the Personal Symptom Checklist (page 141) and please complete it if you haven't already.

The 12 million American women with fibro couldn't possibly feel the same degree and combination of fibro's two most predominant symptoms: pain and fatigue. For this reason, there can simply never be a "one size fits all" approach to treatment. In fact, no two of my fibro patients have ever had identical treatment regimens. Experience has taught me to organize people with fibro into three general groups, each with its own therapy protocol.

After you've recorded your own numbers, see which fibro severity category best describes you. I've also included a few notes regarding your path to getting better. A final note: each one of you, regardless of fibro severity, will benefit from a close reading of the Nearly Natural Cure (page 103).

Mild Fibromyalgia

Muscle pain level 1-4, Fatigue level 1-4

You've come to realize that the symptoms now diagnosed as fibro have been around for about a year. It was only when you felt achy every day that you first thought about going to your MD or chiropractor. You'd been reading articles about fibro, or you saw the Lyrica ads on TV and thought "That sounds like what I have." Maybe it was you who suggested the diagnosis to your doctor rather than the reverse.

Your muscles do hurt, but a hot bath or a good massage

provides considerable relief. For quite awhile now, with this pain and tiredness, you thought you were just getting old. Now that you know it's fibro you're a little worried, but also relieved there's a name for what you've been experiencing. It wasn't all in your head.

Your fibro is probably mild, and I'll reassure you there's an excellent chance you can walk away from it with minimal use of prescription drugs (or without them at all). In fact, you might want to turn directly to the Nearly Natural Cure on (page 103). It's tailor-made for you.

Moderate Fibromyalgia

Muscle pain level 4-7, Fatigue level 4-7

When you look back on it, you've had some muscle pain somewhere for years. It may have begun as carrying stress in your neck and back, but during the past year or so, this pain has spread and become so severe it's begun to interfere with your life. You're feeling tired and achy every morning, old and decrepit when you clamber out of bed. Fortunately, a hot bath or shower still loosens up your muscles and a massage helps temporarily, but you feel you're losing ground. You're tired at the very start of the day. Coffee helps, and you're able to make it almost through your workday, though it takes some effort.

In the afternoons, though, you feel like crashing and the thought of going out in the evening isn't remotely appealing. You count the days to the weekend, when you can do nothing. That stress in your neck and upper back? Your significant other, trying to massage you, remarks your muscles feel like they're encased in cement.

Although you'll get some real relief from the Nearly Natural

Cure (page 103) and I recommend you start it now, for a complete turnaround you'll likely need a little help from prescription medications. That shouldn't stop you from trying the six-week plan, however. A balanced approach of both conventional and alternative therapies may be ideal. You really (really!) need consistent pain relief to get you out of this rut.

To extricate yourself from this pain-stress-fatigue-more pain fibro cycle, you'd likely be using:

- The nutritional supplements outlined in the Nearly Natural Cure and/or one of the three FDA-approved meds for fibro (see Medications for Fibro: How They Work and How They Can Help, page 187).

- A pain medication (see Pain Drugs for Fibro, page 227).

- One or more complementary therapies, such as chiropractic, acupuncture, myofascial release, meditation, and guided imagery (see Alternative Medicine for Fibromyalgia, page 245).

- A few sessions with a therapist if you think significant biographical issues have contributed to your fibro. Read Memories in Your Muscles (page 57) for more on this.

As you improve, as you inevitably will, you'll be able to lower the doses of prescription medications, including pain drugs, and work toward eliminating them altogether. If needed, you can then start the nutritional supplements in the Nearly Natural Cure.

Severe Fibromyalgia
Muscle pain level 7-10, Fatigue level 7-10
You know who you are. You've forgotten what it's like to be

pain-free. Your pain began years ago—five years, ten, you're not even sure anymore. During most of this apparent eternity of pain, doctors endlessly told you there was nothing wrong with you, that your tests were normal, or that you were "just depressed." Your friends and family said, "But you don't look sick." Your ex-husband and his divorce attorney said you were faking it for more money. You were denied disability benefits because the insurance company said there was no such thing as fibro. If you lost your job and health insurance, the same insurance company denied your application for health insurance because your fibro was a "pre-existing condition."

When you finally learned that you had fibro, you may have been told that nothing could be done, or to "just exercise," except, of course, you barely have the energy to make coffee in the morning.

Muscle pain dominates your life. When you touch your muscles, they feel both tender and swollen. You drag your achy body through the day wondering how you'll have the energy for food shopping and preparing dinner. When you watch TV, you have trouble following the story line. Trying to balance a checkbook is like doing complex math. You can't find a comfortable position in bed and you sleep poorly, waking exhausted. You realize your grandmother lived to be 96. You're 45 and feel despondent that this could be your life for the next 50 years.

For you, there's simply no way to reverse this hell without prescription medications. If you have some sort of personal ideology against prescription drugs, you need to process that and overcome it. Because to feel better again you'll need them. Not forever, but initially to breach the high hurdles of your severe fibro.

You'll likely need a combination of the following:

- One (or possibly a combination of two) of the FDA-approved fibro medications (see Medications for Fibro: How They Work and How They Can Help, page 187).

- Adequate pain medication (see Pain Drugs for Fibro, page 227).

- A muscle relaxant (see Other helpful fibro medicines, page 219).

- Probably medication for restful sleep and to improve energy (see Other helpful fibro medicines, page 212).

- A few sessions with a therapist, if you think significant biographical issues have contributed to your fibro (see Memories in Your Muscles, page 57).

- In time, one or more complementary therapies, such as chiropractic, acupuncture, myofascial release, and relaxation techniques like meditation and guided imagery (see Alternative Medicine for Fibromyalgia, page 245). Know that for some people with severe fibro even gentle bodywork therapies can be painful, so plan to try them once your fibro has stabilized (and not before).

- To accomplish all this, you need to find a physician who understands fibro. For help, see these websites and be sure to give your doctor the Physician's Guide to Fibromyalgia (page 299 and also a printable PDF version at our website, wholehealthchicago.com):

  — www.co-cure.org/Good-Doc.htm (fibromyalgia good doctor list)

  — www.fmaware.org (National Fibromyalgia Association — click on "Healthcare Provider Directory")

You'll be able to combine prescription meds with some of the nutritional supplements from the Nearly Natural Cure. Others from that list can ultimately be used to replace some of your prescription drugs as your fibromyalgia improves. Unless you have especially severe fibromyalgia, it's unlikely you'll need to use prescription meds for the rest of your life.

Our goal from the start is to get your 7-10 pain under control, breaking the escalating stress-pain-more stress-more pain cycle that's spinning out of control and has effectively disabled you.

One important point: Because you're a low-serotonin, chemically sensitive woman, you won't need particularly high doses of any prescription medication, especially the ones prescribed for pain. High doses of pain meds actually work less well than low doses, and they're always accompanied by unacceptable side effects. Low doses of pain meds are best. It's an unfortunate likelihood that most of your doctors have never offered you pain meds for fibro. That's why you need a knowledgeable physician.

I'd like you to also carefully read to the Nearly Natural Cure (page 103). Not that you'll be starting with supplements like some of your less-affected fibro sisters. But at some point after paring back the fibro drugs, you'll want to understand how supplements work in much he same way as the pharmaceuticals you've left behind. Also, there are many activities in the nearly-natural regimen than can be enormously helpful, including stress-reduction techniques, journaling, and guided imagery.

There's one more group of fibro patients I see as new patients that deserve separate mention

These are women seen by other physicians who have been correctly diagnosed with fibro. In fact, their diagnosis may have been made several years ago. Initially, they were started on a reasonably good program of prescription medications, but the benefits were either minimal or temporary or the side effects were intolerable. Since their physicians were reasonably well-informed about fibro, as the new FDA-approved drugs became available this group was prescribed these medications as well.

Again, same story: either the meds didn't work or you were flattened by side effects and couldn't continue them. As the years passed, your fibro worsened.

When a patient who's experienced all this arrives in my office for her initial visit, she usually opens a list of "failed medications" as long as my arm. I read through her list and know that some of the meds might have worked had they been prescribed at lower (and more tolerable) doses. That means we can consider re-starting them in the future.

What I almost always find missing from the lengthy drug list is a pain medication (I try to hold back my look of exasperation). Here before me is a woman in chronic daily pain with a condition whose Greek name translates to "muscle pain." Researchers now refer to fibro as a pain amplification syndrome, using such descriptive words as "allodynia" (experiencing pain from normally non-painful stimuli), "hyperalgesia" (increased response to any painful stimuli), and the unique "persistence of pain" (why your trigger-point test still hurts the next day).

This is clearly no way for any human being to go through

life and yet she is denied a pain medication.

If this describes you, begin the Nearly Natural Cure (page 103) and most definitely start on a medicine for your pain (see Pain Drugs for Fibro, page 227). This combination actually can improve your symptoms quite quickly.

6

MEMORIES IN YOUR MUSCLES

This chapter may at first appear to have nothing to do with your fibro, but I assure you it does, and in very important ways. In fact, its central theme applies to many chronic medical conditions, and by reading it you may gain a deeper understanding of someone you care about. If you have fibro, you'll end the chapter with a far clearer perspective on why your muscles hurt and how your fibro was triggered. So let's get started…

Vienna, in the first decades of the 20th century, was a stunning place. By general acclaim, Vienna had risen to become the cultural, artistic, musical, diplomatic, and medical capital of Europe. In America, it was a mark of status to tell friends that your physician had been trained in Vienna.

One young physician there, Dr. Wilhelm Reich, became interested in the fledgling specialty of psychiatry, and he couldn't have been in a better place. He met with his future mentor, Dr. Sigmund Freud, who in turn was so impressed by Reich's intelligence and creativity that in 1922—when Reich was just 26—he invited him to become a staff member of his clinic.

A few years later, Reich lost his favored position with Freud because of what was considered at the time to be his "radical therapeutic techniques." How radical? Instead of communicating with patients in a detached way by sitting out of sight behind the fabled couch, Reich shifted his chair to a position where he and his patient could see each other. This was simply unheard of in those early days of psychotherapy. According to Freud's theories, any eye-to-eye contact would inhibit revelations of the dreams and free associations that were needed to explore the emotional depths of the patient.

But as Reich carefully watched his patients he saw what we now call body language—the silent facial expressions, muscle tension, and postures that enhance the way we communicate with each other. Then Reich took an even more radical step.

He actually touched his patients.

To this day, fearing charges of inappropriate behavior, potential liability, or abuse, mental health practitioners of every stripe are endlessly cautioned, "Don't put your hands on your patient. Period."

But Reich, always a pioneer, did. And what he discovered simply amazed him (and has much to tell us about fibro). Patients were tensing their bodies, so much so that their muscles were often rock-hard, with painful knots.

And Reich knew he was on to something.

The unconscious mind and fibro

He'd already learned from Freud how the mind is divided into three separate areas— conscious, preconscious, unconscious—all endlessly communicating with each other. This separation isn't based on brain anatomy, but rather refers to the mental and emotional content of each region. To understand this concept of brain topography, picture an iceberg floating in the sea, only the top 10% visible. Freud named this tip the *conscious* mind. It contains everything you're aware of at the moment: what you see, hear, say, and think. Right now you're reading these words using your conscious mind.

The remaining 90% of this iceberg-mind is out of sight, below water level. Freud named it the *subconscious* mind and divided it into two sections. The part of the iceberg nearest the water is the *preconscious* mind, and represents about 10 to 15% of your subconscious. This section contains information (memories, images, language) that you can access with varying degrees of ease or difficulty. If I say, "Think of an elephant," up pops in your mind an image of an elephant.

On the other hand, that school exam answer you knew all along but couldn't remember the moment you needed it shows that information is not always easy to retrieve from your preconscious. An image of your mom, what you did on your last birthday, what your childhood room looked like, your opinions: these are all floating through your preconscious mind.

Far below the water's surface is your *unconscious* mind, about 80% of the total, which Freud and Reich viewed as containing everything else. Think of it as your psychic "dump box" for deep-seated long-lost memories, urges, anxieties, feelings, and ideas. We regularly "visit" our unconscious mind in our dreams, but otherwise we can't readily access this vast segment. Your unconscious mind is like the Great and Powerful Oz in "The Wizard of Oz," the great motivator in your life, pulling your strings, even though you're totally unaware your strings are being pulled.

To Freud and Reich, everything you've ever seen, felt, or

thought lurks in your unconscious mind and exerts an influence on actions every day of your life. If I were to ask you, "Why in heaven's name did you marry someone so wrong for you?" you'd come up with a nice logical answer from your preconscious mind. The real reason is hidden deeply in your unconscious, likely connected to relationships with your father, boys in grammar school, hidden issues with self esteem—the list can go on and on. Your unconscious mind is rich and deep.

There are times when your preconscious mind can't come up with an answer at all. "Why are you holding your jaw muscles so tightly?" or "Why do you smile constantly, even when we're talking about something sad?" You might say, "I don't know," or "I didn't know I was doing that," or even "I'm *not* holding my jaw muscles tightly!" "I'm *not* smiling." The answers are beyond your immediate preconscious reach, but explorations into your unconscious mind might reveal answers that would surprise and shock you.

Reich observed how a patient tightened her neck and back muscles or clenched her jaw when a stressful topic came up. He used his hands to actually feel the remarkable tension in these muscles and concluded, in his book *Character Analysis*, that the real cause of this tension lay deeply buried in his patient's unconscious mind.

Your memory palace

Within our remarkable brains, we probably remember everything that's ever happened to us. Picture your mind as a vast fairy-tale palace with thousands of rooms, within each the scenes and emotions of your biography, the book of experiences that make you *you*.

If you concentrate—really concentrate without any outside

distractions—many scenes from childhood will open before you. Delve deeply into one particular room from your childhood to recall small details, like textures, colors, and smells.

One of the most remarkable memory feats in literature was that of French author Marcel Proust, lying in his bed in a cork-lined room, trying to record his life in one of the greatest novels of the 20th century, *Remembrance of Things Past* (or more literally from the French, *In Search of Lost Time*). His evocative recollections include one of the most famous: lifting a morsel of scallop-shelled madeleine pastry dipped in tea to his lips and the flood of childhood memory it released, an "exquisite pleasure" in his own words.

The late historian and essayist Tony Judt, slowly dying of amyotrophic lateral sclerosis (Lou Gehrig's disease) in 2010 and virtually trapped in his paralyzed body, lay awake each night remembering long-lost details of his childhood and youth—the smells of a city bus, the facial expression of an old woman at a candy store when he was six years old and given a few pennies for sweets.

In the 1940s, certain operations on the brain needed to be done with the patient only very lightly sedated. Neurosurgeons quickly discovered that with minimal stimulation of brain tissue, the patient would suddenly "see" a place from her past and, for example, start naming aloud who was gathered around a dining room table. The surgeons had unlocked a room of her memory palace.

In our own palaces, most rooms are darkened, their contents buried deep in the unconscious mind. To a large extent this is a good thing. A lot of these rooms you really don't need to recapture Proustian-style, filled as they are with the insignificant stuff of life. Moreover, if memory were like a

61

David Edelberg, MD

huge TV with all the channels going at once, you'd never manage to get anything done. When this happens with technology — phone, internet cruising, e-mail, Facebook — we call it overload.

Imprinted trauma: how muscles remember everything
Other rooms in the palace of your past are sealed off because your mind simply can't cope with their bad associations — unpleasant events you'd simply rather not recall. The very worst of these traumatic imprints, as Reich called them, are worth pondering not necessarily because they apply to your own biography and fibro, but because they clarify how fibro comes about in the 25% of women who were psychologically, physically, or sexually abused as children or sexually assaulted (date rape) as young women.

What Reich believed was that, along with your brain, your muscles remember everything. On the relatively mild side, your muscles remember a relatively minor physical injury. On the more severe end, repressed memories of emotional trauma are also imprinted and stored in your muscles.

When we actually experience the traumatic event, much of it is simply intolerable to our conscious minds and so we involuntarily force it deep into our unconsciousness. You might vaguely remember having a "dysfunctional childhood," but the details (important details if you have fibro) are lost. You might even say "I can't remember a thing about my childhood!"

Keep in mind that because we're all unique human beings, what constitutes an imprinted trauma can vary widely. A nagging mother insisting her seven-year-old daughter weigh herself twice daily so she doesn't get fat might produce adult depression, body image issues, and an eating disorder in one person and cause minimal psychological damage to another. But psychiatrists and psychologists agree that along with our unique brain chemistries and genetics, traumatic imprints lie at the heart of chronic depression, anxiety, panic attacks, obsessive thinking, and a variety of physical symptoms, including fibromyalgia.

Interestingly, although most imprinted traumas begin with emotionally painful events, they can originate in more extreme physical trauma as well. Consider, for example, a woman we'll call Ann who had a severe car-crash whiplash injury some years ago. Ann tells her doctor she has neck and back pain "that never went away after the crash." Because of her normal x rays and MRI scans there are no positive test results for this muscle pain. Ann may even be eyed with suspicion by her insurance company, suspecting she's faking pain for monetary gain.

In actual fact, the traumatic event of the car accident is now deep in Ann's unconscious mind, which in turn holds her neck and back muscles tight in a valiant but misguided attempt to protect her.

When I gave a talk on fibro and its relationship to childhood abuse to a group of family physicians, one interrupted me with, "But many women I've treated with fibro were abused when they were older. A date rape, abuse by their spouse, anything." This was heartening for me—not the message but the person delivering it. I've been facing groups of skeptical physicians ("I don't believe in fibro") for years, and this GP from a small town in the southeast "got it."

I thanked him for his accurate observation and went on to add that, indeed, the triggering stress of fibro could come from emotional trauma (such as abuse of any type at any age), physical trauma (like an injury that won't clear up), or a combination of the two (such as the emotional stress of a chronic illness and the physical stress that can accompany such a condition).

It's safe to say that virtually all situations—from the mild "I carry my stress in my neck and upper back" to the encapsulating suit of muscular armor women with fibro often wear—likely has some degree of biographical component. At some point in your past you unconsciously (but probably understandably) took the phrase "watch your back" too literally, and tightened yours up.

And now, it won't let go.

Character armoring, muscular armoring

Reich used the term "armoring" to describe an unconscious series of maneuvers we all use to deal with our imprinted traumas, those repressed events buried deep in our unconscious. Like a knight's suit of armor, our own armoring is a superficially good protective cover-up, but in the process of armoring ourselves we inadvertently fail to confront the real issues in our lives.

Reich described two forms of armoring:

- **Character armoring is reflected in our personalities.** For example, a patient I'll call Carissa who had a history of traumatic imprints from sexual abuse, unconsciously created character armor that included distrusting all men and a reluctance to emotionally commit herself to a relationship. A child with a learning disability or ADD creates the character armor of becoming the class clown so that no one will notice his academic shortcomings. A young man angry at the world because he was bullied as a child represses his resentment by creating the armor of good cheer even as he tells his therapist about his sadistic classmates.

- **Muscular armoring occurs when we defend against traumatic imprints with constant muscle tension.** When stressed as a young adult, Carissa tensed her shoulders and back just as she did to protect herself from her abuser as a child. Now, her entire body is sheathed in muscle tension. Our angry young man holds his face in a fixed and mirthless smile. Reich couldn't know it at the time, but his description of muscular armoring is a remarkably accurate description of what decades later would be named fibromyalgia.

As someone with fibro, your muscular armoring extends to the thick fibrous tissue called fascia that sheathes every muscle and muscle group. Fascia is one seriously tough tissue. When you eat a steak, you're eating muscle. The unchewable gristle left behind is fascia.

Sadly for fibro patients, fascia has a rich coating of nerve endings, so when your muscles are tight you experience the added discomfort of fascial pain. Unlike muscle, fascial tissues have a poor blood supply, meaning damaged or excessively constricted fascia heals very slowly.

Constricted fascia also impairs adequate blood supply to muscle, and without it your muscles start to hurt. Tightened muscle and fascia can also literally pinch nerves, so that some women with fibro feel numbness and tingling of their hands and feet, or their skin feels especially sensitive or swollen when to an outsider it looks completely normal.

How stressors trigger a fibro flare in your muscles
So susceptible to stress are the muscles of some women with

fibro that relatively minimal stress can trigger a fibro flare. Many women with fibro are extremely chemically sensitive (you know what I'm talking about, don't you?) and their pain increases sharply following exposure to unpleasant smells, certain foods, or even shifts in the weather, especially changes in barometric pressure.

Each of these situations is a real stressor to a person with fibro, but because test results are normal, many patients are written off by their physicians as whining or neurotic.

So let's get back to Wilhelm Reich. By both observing and touching his patients, he discovered they were locking up emotional wounds not only in the darkened rooms of their memories, but in their muscles as well. It generally follows a pattern that many fibro patients understand: the tightness and pain begin in the neck and shoulders and proceed downward.

My fibro patients routinely report "I always carried my stress in my neck and shoulders, but then things started worsening. My arms, my lower back, my hips and pelvis, and last, my knees."

The most painful area of any muscle is called a tender point, the spot where your contracted muscle attaches itself to bone. You can read more about tender points and how they're used to diagnose fibro on pages 25 and 310.

Understand that as a prelude to your fibro, you likely faced an extremely unpleasant and stressful situation that overloaded your coping skills and your stress-buffering serotonin, triggering your body's stress response (the fight-or-flight response). If you think about it for a moment, what you need to fight or flee are your muscles, so you used yours.

When the stressful period was over and your fight-or-flight response shut down, your muscles were supposed to release themselves. But yours didn't. Constant stress means continued muscle contraction. And when muscles remain contracted, they hurt. This is fibro.

Compared to men, women with their low levels of stress-buffering serotonin are especially susceptible to triggering the fight-or-flight response. Stressed working women come home, race through dinner preparation, help their kids with homework, and then ask their partner, "Honey, rub my back. Harder. Go deep, down where those knots are," muscles as hard as cement blocks.

But a guy, with a serotonin stress-buffer four times that of hers (along with the uniquely male psychological skill of compartmentalizing life), comes home from work tired and sometimes grumpy, but generally he throws himself down on the sofa and relaxes, leaving work back at the office, not faced with the endless to-do list women have, not engaged in a woman's non-stop fight-or-flight response.

Fibro and imprinted trauma

Physicians like me who are oriented toward mind-body medicine know that imprinted traumas can produce long-lasting physical symptoms. So at this point, let me suggest something you may not have heard from your current physician: it is very possible that the effects of one or more imprinted traumatic events — physical (like an old injury) or emotional — either in your remote past or as recently as the year before your fibro developed, are now the source of your fibro pain, exhaustion, and chronic fatigue.

This concept is going to require some consideration.

For example, you might say in protest, "Now just wait a minute. I've got fibro but I'm sure I've had a pretty good life. My childhood was fine. No emotional traumatic events and no physical trauma either."

And here I'd agree. Certainly a majority of people with fibro (75%) don't have a lurking childhood history of sexual abuse responsible now for their chronic daily pain, though many of my patients did grow up in families where anger, alcoholism, or other such stressors dominated life.

Virtually all fibro patients I've worked with report an extended period of unchecked stress before their fibro began. I'm suggesting that your unique response of first carrying your stress in your neck and back, and then tightening up all your muscles, is an unconscious strategy you "learned" when you were younger.

It's essential to appreciate that each of us responds differently to stress. Men rely on their robust amounts of serotonin to keep stressful events from entering their unconsciousness and stirring up trouble. But if you're on the low end of the serotonin curve (female, with a family history of low-serotonin disorders — see page 23), you're highly vulnerable to stress.

This means that a relatively minor trauma — an unkind word from your husband or boss, an unsympathetic doctor, an abrupt change in barometric pressure, exposure to unpleasant-smelling chemicals, or the drop in estrogen during PMS days — can trigger some pretty unpleasant symptoms, like depression, anxiety, or a variety of muscle-tightening symptoms like headache, jaw clenching, or a worsening of your fibro.

"Wait" you might respond. "You're losing me here. What

exactly is the connection between my chemical sensitivity, my fibro, and my nasty alcoholic father?"

Okay, here goes:

- Your sensitivity to chemicals, barometric pressure, or PMS is genetic and all part of your really low stress-buffering system. Your body perceives stressors (smell of chemicals, father's rages, hormone changes) with the same fight-or-flight response you'd experience if a mugger were chasing you: a burst of the hormones adrenalin, norepinephrine, and cortisol.

- These hormones place you into temporary overdrive so you can escape the stress, only in your case it's not a mugger. So instead of escaping the shift in weather or your hormone fluctuations, your muscles tighten up (headaches, jaw clenching) and your heart races (anxiety, panic) until the system exhausts itself (depression, deep fatigue). Perhaps in your particular case as a child whenever you were frightened you tightened your shoulders and your upper back.

- Decades later, your low-serotonin body is responding like the little girl who tensed her body when stressed. Now, confronted with a minor stressor that the men around you don't even notice (chemical smells, change in weather), you experience a full-blown stress response and debilitating flares of fibro and fatigue.

Here's a troubling example from that awful, documented fact: 25% of fibromyalgia adults were emotionally, physically or sexually abused as children. This may not be you at all, but your fibro is a variation on this theme, since the process of protecting yourself from imprinted trauma is the same.

? could the N/V be the stressor that caused the fibro? Or was it an early symptom of fibro?

Remember Carissa? At 38, she's in therapy for chronic depression. She also has all the symptoms of fibro but hasn't reported them to her therapist. She did tell her internist she was constantly tired and achy and he reassured her that all her tests were normal, and that her symptoms were common with depression. He advised her to simply continue her therapy.

Carissa tells her therapist that her biological father left home when she was about eight years old. She doesn't remember him. Her mother started dating and one of the new boyfriends forced himself sexually on Carissa when her mother wasn't home, warning her that he'd would hurt her baby brother if she told anybody and assuring her that all good girls did this. A year later, he's gone from the scene and Carissa never tells her mother what occurred.

For years Carissa rarely thinks about her abuser, the details of what occurred when she was eight relegated to imprinted trauma deep in her unconscious. One of her memory palace rooms, locked tightly. But her intuition makes the connection between her vague recollections of past abuse and her lifelong predisposition to depression, and this prompts her to seek therapy.

Even though the actual events seem lost, "memories" of the stress continue on in her muscles. Carissa had long ago forgotten how she tensed her body, tightened her shoulders, and hunched forward whenever she heard her abuser's key in the door—the fight-or-flight response expressing itself in an eight-year-old girl.

As she learns about more herself in psychotherapy, she realizes she's always carried stress in her neck and upper back. During her twenties when she had that real jerk of a boyfriend, she remembers how a relatively minor argument would cause her whole body to tense up or trigger a nauseating headache. That's when she started wearing a mouth guard, and she still grinds through them at a rate of two or three every year.

Now an adult, Carissa has been reading more about the lifetime health problems linked to childhood abuse. She starts therapy with a psychologist skilled in this field. So far, very good. But the big question remains: does her therapist know of the child abuse-fibro connection so she can make a referral for additional help? Unfortunately, most therapists are ignorant of this, and we'll discuss it more below.

So, here's you, developing fibromyalgia

To briefly reiterate the genesis of your fibro:

- **Genetically you are a low-serotonin woman**, which makes you biochemically much more susceptible to stress than virtually all men and most other women.

- **Because of your low serotonin stress buffer**, you're also more susceptible to one or more of the other low-serotonin fibromyalgia-related disorders. These include depression, anxiety with or without panic attacks, obsessive thinking, compulsive behavior tendencies, eating disorders, social anxiety, post traumatic stress disorder, and seasonal affective disorder. As a consequence, your physical symptoms (in addition to fibro) might include tension and migraine headaches, TMJ, irritable bowel syndrome, PMS, and chronic fatigue (due to adrenal and/or thyroid fatigue). You might instinctively try to treat yourself by eating a lot of carbs or compulsively exercising (both raise serotonin) or using alcohol or other recreational drugs in an attempt to reduce stress. Researchers call fibro a "pain amplification and pain persistence syndrome." This means *you feel pain much more strongly than other people.* If you and a non-fibro friend both are given the same painful irritation (inflating a blood pressure cuff, for example), you'll feel much more discomfort than your friend and your pain will last much longer.

- **Somewhere in your biography you learned to activate your fight-or-flight response by tensing your muscles whenever you were under stress.** You might have learned this as a child in your dysfunctional home. You might have learned it the year or two before you were diagnosed with fibro during that perfect storm of stress—created by job, family, money problems, grief, the list goes on. You might have started tightening your muscles after a sports injury, physical assault, auto accident, or during your years commuting for hours in stop-start expressway traffic.

- **You seek relief to no avail.** To treat your symptoms, you began with massage or chiropractic, mainly because the blood tests and x rays from your family doctor were always negative and you were told nothing was wrong. Unfortunately, the relief from your chiropractor or massage therapist lasted only a day or two, or until you ran out of insurance benefits, money, or both. Over the years, your pain spread. Your tests are still negative, your doctor may have lost interest, and you feel a sense of despair and abandonment. As you'll read in the chapter You've Got A Friend (page 259), which includes details of a survey of 500 women with fibro, at least you'll know you're not alone with these feelings. Small consolation.

Healing emotional wounds

For all women with fibro (and especially those with traumatic childhoods of any stripe), part of getting well — part of breaking this painful cycle of stress/pain and pain/stress — involves healing the emotional wounds that have been partly masked by muscular armoring.

Ironically, if your muscles could talk, they'd say they "meant well" whenever it was they began protecting you in a suit of muscle armor. But with an insufficient serotonin stress-buffering system they over-reacted, remained locked up, and continue to tense themselves further whenever you're exposed to stress.

The first step in healing your fibro asks that you explore your biography. Turn on the light in the darkened rooms of *you* and confront whatever the dazzling brightness reveals.

Keep in mind that whatever stress triggered your fibro may have been more recent, say a year with an abusive partner, job stress, anxiety about the care of your aging parents.

If you can complete the sentence, "I'm pretty sure my fibro began when..." you're taking the first steps toward healing. Ultimately, a few sessions with a therapist might help change your perspective on whatever occurred and lead you to problem-solving clarity instead of locking yourself behind a painful muscle wall.

As you take control of your stressors, you'll realize your muscles aren't hurting as much. This is all part of the Nearly Natural Cure you'll find in page 103.

**Fibro Quicksand: Extensively worrying
about your fibromyalgia**

Educating yourself about fibro (you bought this book—cong-ratulations!) is helpful, but excessive focus on its challenges will only increase your emotional stress, which will in turn worsen your fibro.

Use the tools in this book—healthful eating, stress review, journaling, myofascial release, massage, exercise, talk therapy, supplements and/or medication—to get your pain and energy under control, taking positive steps to structure a life you can handle.

If you have larger worries, let me reassure you about a few fibro facts. No one has ever died of it and none of my patients has been permanently disabled by it. Taken in the doses I recommend, current medications are safe and have no long-term side effects (plus, you'll be reducing your dose and getting off them altogether at some point).

Begin taking the positive steps toward better health outlined in the Fibro-Friendly Eating Plan (page 145) and the Nearly Natural Cure (page 103). Then, begin with the Week 1 assignments.

You'll feel better for having simply moved forward.

Unlocking your darkest rooms with emotional myofascial release therapy

For my fibro patients with deeply rooted emotional issues, the process of unwinding muscles and releasing their trapped memories is made easier with help. A growing number of bodywork therapists are teaming with psychologists to fast-forward the healing process. They do so by manually "opening" your painfully blocked fibro muscles and accompanying you as you light your darkest rooms.

One such field is emotional myofascial release therapy. Many of its practitioners are familiar with Reich and the concept of muscular armoring. The "release" involves muscle, fascia, and blocked memories. If you're among the 25% of people with fibro and a history of an abusive childhood home or a sexual attack at any age, seriously consider emotional myofascial release therapy. Even if you've had psychotherapy to deal with these issues, if your muscles remain in painful knots take it as a signal from your body telling you there's more work to be done.

I first witnessed emotional myofascial release therapy in a fibro patient many years ago. I'd been invited to sit in on a session conducted by a married couple, both therapists, who limited their practice to this challenging but professionally rewarding field. Their patients were virtually all women, though they'd seen a few men as well. Patients had been referred by psychologists, support groups, and other patients who had experienced lasting benefits.

They used a combination of deep tissue massage, muscle stretching, and counseling in a completely safe setting — quiet room, dim lights, low voices — to reverse the muscle armoring. As they gently coaxed muscles, dark rooms lit up too, exposing old wounds. And while the treatment can be emotionally wrenching, it's healthier to confront trauma than to let it fester beneath a muscle-and-fascia straightjacket.

The therapists I quietly watched placed their patient in different positions — lying first on her back, then her stomach, and last curled into a ball — trying to recreate a position her body might have assumed when her muscles began locking up. She now was on her left side, curled into a fetal position, the hands of the therapists kneading her muscles, stroking her hair, speaking in low soothing tones. Suddenly she shouted a horrific scream, rolled off the table, threw herself blindly into one corner of the small room and curled herself up, her body wracked by loud sobs and animal moans. I had never seen or heard anything quite like it. Had she unconsciously recreated the position she'd been in as a child, cowering from an attacker, dodging his blows?

The moment startled me so much I felt my heart pounding, my mouth dry up, my eyes fill with tears. The therapists then positioned themselves on both sides of her, whispered into her ears, gently stroked and hugged her. She wrapped her arms around the woman and continued crying until she lay back exhausted. They signaled me to leave the room, spent another half hour with her, and then she quietly left the office. Afterwards, they told me I'd been fortunate to witness an actual breakthrough. Their patient had been visiting them for weeks and though they knew they were on to something, this had been the session they were hoping for.

Some months later I learned their patient no longer needed the emotional myofascial release therapy and was in a support group of abuse survivors, her path to healing cleared by the therapy I'd witnessed.

The lifetime health consequences of abuse

Fortunately, more and more physicians now recognize the health and psychological risks of being raised in an abusive home. It certainly wasn't always like this. When Freud began working with children, his work summarized in *Three Essays on the Theory of Sexuality*, he himself could not accept these children were having sexual relations of any kind and wrote of their "sexual fantasies." From a 21st century perspective, we now think Freud was interviewing sexually abused children.

A number of books during recent years have generated widespread interest and intelligent therapies for survivors of abuse and trauma. Most cities have one or more support groups. In July, 2010, the journal *Mayo Clinic Proceedings* reported the results of a vast review of psychiatric literature from 1980 through 2008, concluding what many had suspected. Sexual abuse was associated with a lifetime risk of disorders including depression, anxiety, eating disorders, sleep disorders, post-traumatic stress disorder, and suicide attempts. The risks went even higher when there was a history of rape.

In October, 2009, the journal *Headache* reported that a history of child abuse was significantly associated with chronic pain conditions including headache and fibro. A total of 1,348 patients attending a headache clinic were asked to complete a 28-item questionnaire that measured physical, sexual, and emotional child abuse, physical and emotional neglect, and also whether they had, along with their headaches, been diagnosed with fibro, chronic pelvic pain (or interstitial cystitis), chronic fatigue syndrome, or irritable bowel syndrome. The number of different forms of childhood abuse correlated with the number of chronic pain conditions in adulthood.

In the study, 40% suffered chronic headaches and 38% had been abused as children (21% physical abuse, 25% sexual abuse, 38% emotional abuse, 22% physical neglect, 38% emotional neglect). Multiple forms of abuse and neglect were associated with an increasing number of chronic pain conditions. At the time of the study, 28% of the patients were being treated for depression, 56% for anxiety. Abuse issues were "substantially higher in women than in men." These patients also had one predictable laboratory abnormality: a "sluggish response to adrenal stimulation by the pituitary gland." As you'll discover in this book, this is a description of adrenal fatigue.

Your mind and body are inseparable

Here's something that should cause women around the world to sit up and take notice: tens of millions of women are currently suffering a smorgasbord of low-serotonin, stress-related conditions (called the fibromyalgia spectrum) and nearly 40% have their origins in childhood. Psychiatrist Linda Carpenter, MD, from Alpert Medical School at Brown University in Rhode Island, believes pediatricians should do more and better screening for evidence of abuse now that we know of the lifetime health consequences. She's uncertain what to do about adult women in chronic pain, saying "it is not clear that doctors should do anything differently as a consequence of this finding, but awareness may impact the way we speak with or examine our patients as well as the treatments we offer them."

Although I was pleased that these articles were published, it's going to be slow going. When I recently attended a fibro meeting whose purpose was to introduce the new FDA-approved fibro drug Savella, I asked the physician who had conducted Savella's clinical trials, "Do you routinely bring up the childhood abuse issue among the hundreds of patients enrolled in your study?"

He looked very uncomfortable at this question, lowered his voice and literally stammered out, "No, we don't do that. We never do unless they bring it up. If they do, we refer them to psychiatrists."

I definitely did not like that response, and probably couldn't conceal my sneer-scowl of displeasure. We as physicians are responsible for the health and well-being of the whole person, emotional and physical health together as a single entity. Fibro is the ultimate mind-body disorder and to focus solely on mind or body, and pass the buck on the other, will lead nowhere.

Fortunately there's a steadily growing group of physicians who recognize this connection and devote their practice to the whole person: the American Holistic Medical Association (AHMA). If there were any physician who would immediately explore your biography as it related to biology of your fibro, it would be a member of the AHMA.

The AHMA's membership is well under a thousand physicians, but there are members in every state. Considering there are about 750,000 doctors currently in practice, this is a very small number. The AHMA is the ultimate organization of mind-body medicine and you've got to like an organization whose older members tie their long gray hair into ponytails. They see lots of fibro patients and regularly work with alternative therapies like chiropractors, acupuncturists, and myofascial release therapists.

I myself was first exposed to the connection between child sexual abuse and chronic illness at an AHMA meeting during talks given by Drs. Carolyn Myss and Christiane Northrup. I was genuinely shocked by the data they were presenting. Carolyn's mantra likely affected us all: They key to understanding your patient is to remember that biography controls biology. The biography of your patient is everything.

I'd like you to take this to heart and explore your own biography as it relates to your fibro.

They sell a T-shirt to doctors at AHMA meetings. It reads "Hugs Heal." And for a fibro patient whose biography can bring tears to the eyes of her doctor, sometimes a hug does work best.

Walk away from fibro

In sum, the armoring described by Reich in the 1920s we now know as fibro. Fibro not only distorts muscles, it distorts lives. But for most people fibro is completely curable. Yes, you can walk away from it and get back to your life. It's a rougher path for women whose fibro history runs to decades, but with the help of the counseling, bodywork, nutritional supplements, and medications I lay out for you in the rest of this book, everyone can return to useful and productive lives.

Fibro never turns into another illness, doesn't shorten anyone's lifespan, has never appeared as the cause of death on anyone's death certificate.

But just being fibro is challenge enough.

80

7

TESTS EVERY FIBRO PATIENT
SHOULD KNOW ABOUT

Fibromyalgia is a clinical diagnosis, meaning it's diagnosed by your medical history and physical exam alone, with no lab tests needed. Good thing, too, as there are no tests of any kind—blood, urine, saliva, x-ray, CT, MRI, or biopsy—that will confirm a diagnosis of fibro or any of its related disorders. When doctors order tests, they're making sure nothing else is going on.

And yet as you'll see in this chapter there are laboratory tests that are helpful in showing your genetic susceptibility to fibro as well as revealing the possible causes of your fatigue. While these tests don't actually diagnose fibro, they can guide you and your physician toward the best medications and nutritional supplements for managing symptoms.

These tests are not "alternative medicine" by any means, but many doctors are unaware of their availability, mainly because they were developed by small clinical laboratories with limited advertising budgets and appeared years after your doctor completed his or her professional training. In the general scheme of health care costs, these tests aren't particularly expensive and, if ordered by your doctor, may be covered by health insurance.

The fibromyalgia spectrum

Doctors who have worked with fibro patients for years understand there are numerous conditions associated with it, called the fibromyalgia spectrum. If questioned, just about every person with fibro reports that in addition to fibro pain, she's experienced one or more of the following low-serotonin disorders some time in her life: depression, anxiety, obsessive thinking, compulsive behavior, an eating disorder, seasonal affective disorder, post traumatic stress disorder, tension and/or migraine headaches, irritable bowel syndrome, premenstrual syndrome, chronic fatigue syndrome.

A real spectrum of utter awfulness stealing away life's pleasures and joys.

Setting aside mood disorders (including depression and anxiety), let's talk about the physical conditions on that list. They're called "functional" conditions by physicians because they're not viewed as manifestations of disease, but rather as a problem with the way your body functions.

Another doctor term for them is somatoform disorders, "soma" being the Greek word for body. At one time, somatoform disorders were the Rodney Dangerfields of medicine, getting no respect from physicians. However, as doctors became more aware of the impact functional disorders had on their patients' lives, somatoform/functional disorders began to get a little more attention.

Here are some recent statistics: If we add up all the people coming to medical offices for any of the non mood disorder conditions in the fibro spectrum, the numbers are vast. 25 to 50% of all office visits are due to symptoms of somatic/functional disorders, with an estimated total of 400 million clinic visits a year. The vast majority of visits to certain specialists are due to somatoform disorders. Chronic headaches are the mainstay of neurologists and I'd guess half a gastroenterologist's practice deals with irritable bowel syndrome.

Add in the psychological symptoms and mood disorders, primarily depression and anxiety, and the numbers are staggering.

In 2010, the highly respected *American Journal of Medicine* published an extensive review of all available literature on somatoform disorders, focusing on depression, fibro, and irritable bowel syndrome (IBS) in an attempt to amass and make sense of some of the data that had been accumulating.

If you've been following me thus far, there will be no surprises in these, the report's main conclusions:

- Depression, fibro, and irritable bowel syndrome (IBS) routinely overlapped each other, meaning if you had one you were likely to have one or both of the others.

- At any time, 10 to 15% of the general population reports widespread muscle pain (fibromyalgia) and this group was three times more likely to report depression than those without pain. Since fibro affects 95% women, you need to double those numbers to get an accurate idea of how many women are affected—20 to 30% of all women are affected by one or more somatoform disorders.

- The onset of chronic pain was typically associated with poor mental and physical health quality of life (what we'd call stress).

- IBS was strongly linked with widespread pain,

depression, and anxiety.

- Fibro, IBS, and depression run in families, with heritability among females estimated at 50%, meaning that half your girl offspring will likely have one of these if you do.

- Although a specific gene has yet to be identified, the main defect in the three disorders appears to center on the production or utilization of serotonin and other neurotransmitters (brain chemicals).

- People with depression, fibro, or IBS have an exaggerated immune response. If we envision serotonin as a stress buffer, people with these disorders have a lower buffer and as a consequence their immune systems "overreact" to otherwise harmless stimulation. This produces a phenomenon called central sensitization, which causes nerve pain fibers to fire constantly. Relatively innocuous stressors (such as weather changes or certain foods) can trigger pain fibers to fire.

- Not only do these patients feel pain more than others, but they can't turn off the pain once it starts. This phenomenon can occur both in muscles (fibro) and intestines (IBS).

- One part of the stress response system—called the hypothalamic-pituitary-adrenal axis (HPA axis)—is abnormal in people with fibro, chronic fatigue, depression, and IBS. Fibro patients are unable to release adequate amounts of the adrenal hormone cortisol in response to stressors (a fancy definition of adrenal fatigue).

With information like this culled from thousands of patients, a much clearer picture of the fibro spectrum is drawn.

Now let's talk about what tests are available

When I'm working with a fibro patient (or someone with any of the fibro spectrum disorders), I order these tests:

1. Neurotransmitter profile
2. Adrenal hormone profile
3. Thyroid profile with basal body temperature thyroid testing
4. Food sensitivity profile with separate gluten sensitivity testing
5. Vitamin D

I'll discuss each in detail below.

1. Neurotransmitter (brain chemicals) profile

Every doctor in the US was taught in medical school that serotonin is not measurable, but this isn't true. Things have changed.

When depressed patients are prescribed one of the numerous serotonin-raising antidepressant meds, many ask how it works. Psychiatrists answer, "It increases brain levels of your neurotransmitter serotonin." Some patients then ask, "Can we run a test to see how low my serotonin actually is?" And virtually every psychiatrist in the country will answer, "No."

Not only is this incorrect, but many people reluctant to start an antidepressant for whatever reason might be more inclined to do so if they could see exactly how low their serotonin level was.

This has all been frustrating for Dr. Gottfried Friedlander, who some years ago developed techniques for measuring neurotransmitters and then founded NeuroScience Inc in Osceola, Wisconsin. (Recently neuroScience was acquired by

Pharmasan Labs, a huge specialty testing company whose main customer is the Mayo Clinic.)

I sat down with Dr. Friedlander to discuss this issue. "It is so frustrating trying to change the thinking of doctors," he said. "They learn 'you can't measure serotonin' and when you show them that you can, and show them the results, they shake their heads and say it can't be done."

His encounter with psychiatrists reminded me of how, in 1830, engineers from France crossed the English Channel for the first ever demonstration of a train moving under its own power (steam, as opposed to horse drawn). They road the rails back and forth, returned to France, and reported to the government that steam-driven trains were "impossible." There had to have been a trick.

The test that measures neurotransmitters is simplicity itself (Pharmasan also offers a more elaborate test, checking additional neurotransmitters, but this isn't necessary). You receive a kit containing a plastic vial for your urine. On a morning you choose, you wake up and urinate into the toilet. Then, eating and drinking nothing, you wait until you have to pee again. That's the one you collect. Urinate into the vial, mail it to the lab. Done.

Here's what gets measured and how to interpret the results:

1. Norepinephrine
2. Epinephrine
3. Dopamine
4. Serotonin
5. GABA
6. Creatinine

First consider norepinephrine and epinephrine. These two neurotransmitters are primarily stored in the stress-responding adrenal medulla of your adrenal glands (more on them in #2 below). Under stress, levels of both norepinephrine and epinephrine increase, putting you into temporary overdrive. If you constantly flog your adrenals with stress (hallmark of fibro), the glands become "fatigued" and these levels drop. Low levels of epinephrine and norepinephrine indicate exhausted adrenal glands...and an exhausted you.

Dopamine is low (but not consistently low) in people who have attention deficit disorder or Parkinson's disease. When you're in love, your dopamine levels are very high.

Serotonin you've heard a great deal about already. It's the feel-good neurotransmitter that also acts as a buffer against stress.

GABA (gamma amino butyric acid) is low in people with anxiety disorders. GABA is actually sold as a safe and effective nutritional supplement for anxiety.

Creatinine is not a neurotransmitter at all. It comes from muscles and is measured to ensure you've provided a suitable urine specimen.

In a typical patient with fibro or any of its related disorders, I expect to find a low serotonin stress buffer and also low epinephrine and norepinephrine, reflecting adrenal fatigue. However, I've certainly had a few patients with fibro who had normal levels of serotonin. So many factors can affect serotonin (most notably antidepressant medications, which boost levels) that I don't use low serotonin levels alone to make a fibro diagnosis. Rather, this measurement is helpful in showing you your susceptibility to stress.

I always explain to my patients that low serotonin is genetic (something else you can blame your parents for, start an argument about, and ruin another Thanksgiving dinner).

2. Adrenal Hormone Profile

They're about the size of walnuts, your two adrenal glands. Picture them resting comfortably, one on top of each kidney. If you place your hands on your hips and extend your thumbs, your thumbs are pressing at the location of your adrenal glands. Receiving signals from two separate parts of your brain, the adrenals put you into overdrive when you're confronted with stress.

There are two parts to your adrenals: inner (medulla) and outer (cortex).

- **The adrenal medulla** responds to emergency signals from your brain, releasing neurotransmitters that put your whole body into emergency super-high gear. When you read about a 90-year-old woman beating back a mugger with her umbrella, you can be sure she has an enviable pair of adrenals.

  The medulla is directly connected to your brain—it's actually considered part of your nervous system rather than part of your endocrine (glandular) system. When stimulated by a sudden stress like the mugger or an oncoming vehicle it releases epinephrine (adrenaline) and norepinephrine, which speed up heart rate, raise blood pressure, and enhance breathing and other overdrive necessities.

- **The adrenal cortex** responds to long-term stress, producing DHEA (a pre-hormone that makes other hormones), cortisol, and the sex hormones progesterone and testosterone. It is an actual gland, like your thyroid and ovaries. The adrenal cortex is under the control of your master gland, the pituitary, a small but potent nugget tucked beneath your brain.

The stress response of the adrenal cortex is slower and more sustained. Instead of a quick jolt to your adrenal medulla, this stress message is relayed deep into an area of your brain called the hypothalamus, which sends the signal on to your pituitary, which in turn activates the adrenal cortex to release a variety of hormones, the most important being cortisol. This pathway is called the "hypothalamic-pituitary-adrenal axis" (HPA axis, for short) and dysfunction of the HPA is a well-recognized phenomenon in fibro, depression, irritable bowel syndrome, and chronic fatigue syndrome.

Cortisol acts more subtly than epinephrine and has effects on blood sugar metabolism, immunity, energy, and inflammation. During prolonged stress, your adrenal cortex produces excess cortisol, which, while doing some good things to bail you out of your crisis, can also trigger weight gain, especially around your abdomen, and interfere with focus and concentration.

With protracted stress, your adrenal cortex can become fatigued and slow to respond to messages from the pituitary. It was shown some years ago that the adrenal glands of chronic fatigue and fibro patients responded sluggishly to pituitary stimulation. The test for this sluggish response is complex and cumbersome, involving injecting pituitary hormones and then measuring blood levels of cortisol.

Far easier is a simple adrenal hormone test kit prepared by Pharmasan (and several other companies) using timed collections of saliva over a single day. Your cortisol levels normally start out on the high side in the morning, slowly declining as the day progresses. They're lowest at bedtime and then, as you sleep, cortisol levels are restored, like a battery charging up at night.

The adrenal hormone test kit contains four plastic vials with instructions to collect samples at four-hour intervals during a single day. You then mail the specimens back to the lab. Some labs also measure levels of DHEA (dehydroepiandrosterone), a sort of "pre-hormone" or building block for all the other hormones from the adrenals.

I've been puzzled by the reluctance of most endocrinologists to accept that adrenal fatigue exists. They seem to believe that either the adrenals work fine or don't. When they absolutely don't you've got a rare condition called Addison's disease. Endocrinologists generally also have bad things to say about using saliva to test adrenal hormone levels—namely that saliva can't convey the status of hormones as well as blood. However, many research papers have shown that in fact levels of hormones found in saliva are extremely accurate and reliable.

The saliva kits are reasonably priced and most health insurance companies, not caring which fluid a doctor chooses to measure, will reimburse. The number of doctors regularly using salivary testing is in the tens of thousands, not as many as should be.

Thyroid profile with basal body temperature thyroid testing
While the previously mentioned article in the *American Journal of Medicine* discusses the adrenal glands in terms of fatigue, it neglects the thyroid gland, which also goes into overdrive when you're stressed, and the thyroid too can become fatigued.

Here's a short course on the admittedly challenging topic of thyroid hormones, which you need to understand so you can help your doctor diagnose and treat you. As a quick refresher, your thyroid sits in the front part of your neck and acts literally as your body's gas pedal. Too much thyroid hormone output is like placing the clutch of your car in neutral and pressing down on the gas pedal. Too little and everything s-l-o-w-s down.

The main symptoms of too little hormone (low thyroid, or hypothyroidism) are fatigue, cold hands and feet, dry skin and hair, menstrual irregularities and infertility, and weight gain. Hypothyroidism is extremely common, especially among women, and it also seems to run in some families.

Often though, when patients relate these low-thyroid symptoms to their doctors they're told everything is normal because their thyroid blood-test results are normal. If you have the symptoms of an underactive thyroid, understand that low doses of thyroid hormone are a very safe means of restoring you to a normal level. But because doctors are victims of intense pharmaceutical advertising, they often prescribe the second-best treatment: a synthetic hormone instead of the best treatment, an inexpensive, natural one.

Our thyroid glands actually produce two hormones, called thyroxine (T4) and tri-iodothyronine (T3). The synthetic form (Synthroid) contains only T4 and using it assumes your body can convert the T4 to T3, giving you enough of each. Some people are thought to not convert their T4 efficiently. To cover this possibility, using natural thyroid (better known as Armour thyroid), a mixture of both T4 and T3, seems a wise choice.

Thyroid testing

Many physicians, myself included, regard using the standard thyroid test—the TSH (thyroid-stimulating hormone) test—to be notoriously unreliable as a screen for thyroid disorders. There are three reasons for this:

1. TSH is not secreted by the thyroid, but by the gland that controls your thyroid—your pituitary gland, the body's master gland. If your TSH is high, that means your pituitary is sending out a gusher of hormone, trying to flog your low-producing thyroid into making more of its own hormone. A fact that endlessly confuses medical students: *high* TSH means *low* thyroid function. In other words, TSH is an indirect measurement of thyroid function. A more direct measurement would gauge levels of the two actual thyroid hormones, T3 and T4, but this test is rarely done unless TSH levels are abnormal.

2. Even doctors disagree about what level of TSH signals an underactive thyroid. For years, any TSH over 5.0 meant that you had low thyroid and needed treatment. Now, more and more doctors, myself included, believe that any TSH result above 2.5 should be treated with supplementary thyroid hormones. This means that millions of people (mostly women) whose TSH results ranged between 2.5 and 5.0 are living fatigued lives with untreated low thyroid.

3. The unchecked fight-or-flight stress that barrels into the HPA (hypothalamic-pituitary-adrenal/thyroid) axis exhausts the entire system, including the pituitary gland. Even if your pituitary wanted to make more TSH to stimulate your failing thyroid, it can't because it's tuckered out. The result is that your thyroid is underfunctioning *and* your TSH, instead of being high, is

normal or even low. This leads doctors who look mainly at test result numbers (and not as closely at your symptoms) and see a normal or low TSH to conclude your thyroid function is fine.

The result is that women who feel for certain that their thyroids are not making enough hormone endlessly hear from doctors, "I know it seems like your thyroid is underfunctioning. You sure have all the symptoms. But your TSH—it's normal—and I don't prescribe thyroid hormone to anyone with a normal TSH."

This is where basal body temperature testing comes to the rescue.

Do this!

A do-it-yourself low-thyroid test: basal body temperature

What exactly is basal body temperature? "Basal" means "base," and your basal temperature is your body temperature taken the very first thing in the morning before you've moved out of your sleeping position. Once you get out of bed, the movement of your muscles heats up your body, so it's essential that you follow these instructions closely to get an accurate reading.

To take your basal body temperature:

- Use an old-fashioned mercury thermometer or, if your can't find one, buy a digital basal thermometer at any drugstore. These are the same thermometers used for ovulation testing.

- Place the thermometer on your bedside table with paper and pen (if using a mercury thermometer, shake it down before going to sleep).

- When you awaken, place the bulb of the thermometer in your armpit and leave it there for 10 minutes. Lie back and relax, keeping your armpit closed over the thermometer.

- After 10 minutes, record the temperature.

- Repeat for five days and then take an average (you remember this from grade school, right? Add the five numbers and then divide by five to get the average).

- If you're still menstruating, measure your basal body temperature on the second day after your period starts. Ovulation, which occurs later in the month, increases your temperature and thus won't give an accurate reading.

If your average basal temperature is below 97.6, you would likely benefit from a small dose of natural thyroid replacement, usually in the range of one half grain to 1 grain daily, available by prescription, to improve energy. Take the results of your basal body temperature to your physician and explain you'd like to try a small dose of natural thyroid replacement.

Here's a real story about all this thyroid madness

A patient in her mid-30s I'll call Sandra came to our office some time ago and described to me all the classic low-thyroid symptoms: fatigue, cold hands and feet, dry skin and hair, etc. She knew she had thyroid problems, but her previous thyroid tests had revealed nothing. Sandra was also having trouble getting pregnant and had started working with an infertility specialist, moving along the standard infertility treatment treadmill.

Most of Sandra's siblings were taking thyroid hormone and she really wanted to try it before subjecting herself to her second and very expensive infertility treatment (remember, thyroid hormones dramatically affect fertility).

"I told my doctor that I thought I had low thyroid not only because of my symptoms and my sisters, but also because my mom couldn't get pregnant until she started on thyroid, and then she had six of us all in a row." Yet because of Sandra's "normal" TSH results, her doctors had told her that her thyroid was fine.

On hearing about Sandra's mother, my nurse assistant Liz's eyes widened and she said something like, "If Dr. E doesn't write you the thyroid prescription, I will!" Of course Sandra left the office with a thyroid prescription. Six weeks later she sent me an e-mail to let me know she was pregnant (as you might imagine, these e-mails make my day).

If you like stories like this, feel you've been ignored in your quest to try thyroid hormones, or just want to learn more about the thyroid controversy, check out a wonderful website called Stop The Thyroid Madness.

4. Food sensitivity profile with separate gluten sensitivity testing

Except for obvious food allergies, like the severe reactions from peanuts and shellfish or lip swelling from strawberries, I was never taught a thing in medical school about food sensitivities as a cause of chronic illness. And decades later, medical students haven't progressed one iota. Gastroenterologists, allergists, and rheumatologists are either oblivious to the role of toxic foods or openly hostile to the concept.

When I explain the reasons for this deliberate ignorance of food sensitivities to non-medical people they shake their heads in disbelief. They don't believe American physicians would compromise the health of their patients on the basis of nothing more than a glorified turf war.

Here's the story on a controversial diagnosis called "leaky gut." The US medical profession's contempt for any research not homegrown may have played a part in this. The first articles about toxic foods appeared in South African medical journals in the 1960s. More articles then appeared in the UK. American doctors seem to vaguely distrust anything beyond our borders, and woe betide any research that has to be translated.

What South African doctors realized was that certain foods could sufficiently irritate the lining of the intestinal tract so that large, incompletely digested food molecules could "leak" through the intestinal barrier. This, in turn, would trigger an emergency response from the immune system, which would produce antibodies in much the same way that antibodies are produced against viruses, bacteria, and even cancer cells. However, instead of the antibody (called an IgG antibody) clearing out these large food molecules, it instead attached itself to them, and this clump would land somewhere in the body and start causing problems. It might irritate joint linings and produce arthritis symptoms, irritate sinuses and cause chronic nasal congestion, or land in muscles and diminish muscle efficiency, causing fatigue.

This unusual reaction to food differed from regular allergies (like hay fever or hives) because with an allergy, a different family of antibodies (IgE) shows up and triggers the release of the chemical histamine, which causes symptoms. This is why you take an anti-histamine, like Claritin, for hayfever.

Given this information, US allergy specialists stated categorically, "If there's no histamine, there's no allergy. This 'leaky gut' stuff is nonsense!"

Then they convinced the gastroenterologists there were no food sensitivities with comments like "Do antihistamines work for ulcerative colitis? Of course not." Worse yet, the insurance companies, not wanting to pay for anything to begin with, asked the allergists if they should be paying for food sensitivity testing. "Ha!" answered the allergy association, "Why not pay for homeopathy or snake oil or acupuncture while you're at it."

And so, to this day, the vast majority of health insurers will not pay for food sensitivity testing unless (and here's the best part) it is performed under the supervision of a certified allergist and specifically tests for IgE antibodies.

Food sensitivity blood test…and the superior self-test

Several labs offer comprehensive food sensitivity testing using a small sample of blood. The typical profile determines whether or not your immune system is creating antibodies of the IgG class (some labs test for both IgE and IgG) to 96 commonly eaten foods. If antibodies are present, the assumption is that your body doesn't like that food and your immune system is creating antibodies to get rid of it.

Although this food sensitivity profile is a good test, it's not great. It's most useful at revealing a culprit food you may not have suspected was a problem. It fails being great because foods known to be irritating can actually be missed by the test. And you, not knowing this, keep eating the same culprit foods and your immune system continues grinding out antibodies.

The most accurate test for food sensitivities, including gluten, requires no lab at all. It's a do-it-yourself project, described in the Food Sensitivity Elimination-Reintroduction Eating Program (page 167).

Consistently superior to any lab test, it's simple in concept and results: when you eliminate from your diet a food you're sensitive to (such as dairy or gluten) you feel better (less fibro pain, more energy). When you reintroduce the food, your symptoms return.

Currently, millions of people are eating foods that are responsible for a wide range of chronic symptoms, from memory problems and asthma to headaches and obesity. These same people swallow vast amounts of prescription drugs to suppress, but never cure, their symptoms. This of course pleases the pharmaceutical industry, which would collapse if patients started taking their health into their own hands.

But that's precisely what I'd like you to do. Read part three of the Fibro-Friendly Eating Plan (page 164) for a plan to easily test yourself for food sensitivities. Once you complete it, you'll know not only which foods you might be sensitive to, you'll also understand decisively if you need to ask your doctor for a gluten sensitivity test.

5. Vitamin D

Worldwide, there's much new research relating vitamin D to seemingly unrelated medical conditions, among them fibro. A group of doctors in Belfast, Northern Ireland, measured the blood levels of vitamin D in 75 women with fibro. They also administered a questionnaire to determine the degree to which anxiety and depression were part of the symptom list. Here are the results:

- Vitamin D deficiency is extremely common in fibro patients.

- Those with the lowest levels of vitamin D had the most significant anxiety and depression symptoms.

Although the authors made no specific recommendations about using vitamin D for fibro, I suggest the following:

- Take 1,000-2,000 IU of vitamin D daily, especially if your fibro symptoms are accompanied by anxiety and/or depression. If you can convince your doctor to measure your vitamin D level, that would give you an idea of the extent of your possible deficiency.

- Walk in the sunlight, without sunglasses and in short sleeves, for at least 15 minutes a day. Your body makes vitamin D when your skin is exposed to sunlight. To raise your serotonin, you need to "see the sunlight" unobstructed by sunglasses.

Conclusion

Let me summarize briefly how we're going to set about curing your fibro and fatigue based on the information you've learned about these tests. Having the tests themselves is not necessary for successful treatment (although I do ask that all patients take their basal temperature to establish thyroid function).

1. **Because your fibro was triggered by unchecked stress,** working on the stress issues in your life is of paramount importance. You may already feel a little stress relief with my reassurance that your chronic pain, fatigue, and

other symptoms are real and that you're not going crazy. For people with fibro, who are extra-sensitive, sources of stress can include certain foods, hormone imbalance (PMS), and weather-related issues (seasonal affective disorder and barometric pressure changes). As you'll learn elsewhere in this book, other major sources of stress include the pain itself (again, fully treatable) and the stress of facing unsympathetic friends, family, employers, and health care and insurance systems. These stressors are in addition to the all-too-common stress felt by being over-extended, an awful job situation, family drama, and the like.

2. **Your stress-buffering serotonin is inadequate for your needs.** Although your levels are largely genetically predetermined (thanks, mom), you can increase serotonin via exercise, the right foods, and supplements or FDA-approved medications.

3. **As a result of uncontrolled stress, your adrenal glands are fatigued.** This is reflected as inadequate levels of norepinephrine, cortisol, and DHEA. Each of these can be increased, again with either medications or supplements.

4. **Your thyroid is also fatigued** and you may need temporary thyroid hormone replacement.

5. **This whole process is capable of reversing itself** (oh, your awesome human body). Once your stress buffer is stronger, your adrenal and thyroid levels are good, and your pain is under control, most fibro patients can go off or dramatically reduce their pain medications and thyroid and adrenal hormones/supplements. However, because of your genetic low-serotonin stress susceptibility, virtually everyone needs to take

something to maintain healthy and protective serotonin levels, either a medication or nutritional supplement.

6. **If symptoms begin to return, don't panic.** Ask instead: where is my stress coming from?

For more on all this, read the Nearly Natural Cure (page 103).

8

DR E'S SIX-WEEK NEARLY NATURAL FIBRO CURE

This section will help you reverse your fibromyalgia without any prescription drugs. People with fibro are just generally more chemically sensitive, most at some point having experienced at least one nasty side effect that now makes them shrink at the sight of a doctor's prescription pad. I understand. And that's why in this plan you'll be working primarily with herbal and nutritional supplements, body therapies, healthful eating, and stress reduction. Remember that stress triggers and exacerbates fibro. Getting a handle on it is really Job 1.

One very interesting study from Europe showed that simply educating patients about fibromyalgia improved their symptoms. I've seen this in my own practice, the relief on a patient's face when I give her my fibro overview and reassure her nobody's ever died of it. To educate yourself fully, I suggest you finish this book and meditate on your own fibromyalgia for a few days. Then decide which approach — natural or not — you'll undertake.

Based on my experience treating more than 1,600 fibromyalgia patients, those with longstanding symptoms (five or more years of deeply entrenched pain) generally, but certainly not always, need a little help from prescription medicines. That's because their muscles, and the thick fibrous tissue covering them, called fascia, have literally been locked up for years.

Even if you're in this group, you can certainly start this six-week program and move toward supplemental prescription medication at any time. So begin by reading through both this section and the one that follows (What To Do If the Nearly Natural Approach Isn't Working, page 138) and then follow your intuition.

All people with fibromyalgia can benefit from this plan

Whatever your choice, each of you, regardless the status of your fibro, can be helped enormously by following the nutrition, exercise, guided meditation, de-stressing, bodywork, and counseling recommendations in this six-week cure.

If I could be granted one wish for all of you, it would be that your circumstances allowed you to begin your quest for conquering fibro with at least a one-week stay at a residential spa. Here the European health care system shines. In many countries, physicians can refer their fibromyalgia patients for a week of healthful eating, supervised gentle exercise, thermal baths, massage, and educational classes. In a survey given to fibro patients after completing spa therapies, virtually 100% reported "much improvement."

Now of course these patients weren't cured of their fibromyalgia during that week, and when they returned to their stressful lives most symptoms returned as well. But the knowledge they gained about their bodies—how stress exacerbated symptoms, how exercise and massage bring relief—clearly made the spa visit an invaluable lesson in understanding fibro that they could use for the rest of their lives.

Here are the positives and negatives of supplements and prescription medicines:

Advantages of nutritional supplements: Gentle to your body, virtually free of side effects, likely covered by your Health Savings Account if you have one at work.
Disadvantages: May not be strong enough to control your fibro symptoms.

Advantages of prescription medications: Significantly more potent than nutritional supplements. Thus, you're more likely to feel benefits sooner than with supplements.
Disadvantages: Side effects, cost.

Before you dive into the nearly natural cure, let's review exactly who and what we're treating when we treat fibromyalgia:

- **A person, usually a woman,** who is genetically more susceptible to stress because of an inherited low-serotonin stress buffer.

- **Before her fibro started, she likely experienced a protracted period of stress**—emotional or physical—which, due to her body's constant fight-or-flight response, has tightened her muscles painfully and fatigued her stress-responding adrenal glands and thyroid.

- **She now suffers** widespread muscle pain, exhaustion, and unrefreshing sleep.

- **Although the specific triggering events may have receded,** the stress from her current fibro (unrelenting pain, exhaustion, little help from doctors) keeps everything going. In addition, she may have heightened sensitivity to other yet undiscovered but correctable stressors, including diet choices, weather, shifting sex hormones, job, and relationships.

Week 1: Taking Charge of Your Health

This will be a busy week for you as you lay the groundwork for the weeks to come. My suggested time-frame is highly flexible. For example, you may not be able to get an appointment with your doctor for two or three weeks and you may not be able to take your basal temperature until your next menstrual cycle. Use this more as a to-do list rather than a "must do this week or else" list. I'd also like you to read this entire book before starting... and you just might be a slower reader.

1. Make an appointment to confirm your fibro self-diagnosis with your physician...or find a new one. Obviously, if you've already been diagnosed with fibro and you're pleased with your doctor, skip to #2. If you're unfortunate enough to be connected to a physician who "doesn't believe in fibromyalgia" or who hasn't been listening to you for years, it's time to find someone new.

Look for a compassionate doctor who is familiar with fibromyalgia, understands mind-body connections, and is open to using alternative therapies like chiropractic and Chinese medicine (page 245). He or she should be willing to write prescriptions for physical therapy, myofascial release therapy, and massage so that your health insurance can offset some of your expenses. It's essential that your doctor be a full partner in your treatment. For more, read Ask Dr E:

How Should I Prepare for My Doctor Visit? (page 111).

To locate doctors specializing in fibro, check these websites
www.co-cure.org/Good-Doc.htm (fibromyalgia good doctor list)
www.fmaware.org (National Fibromyalgia Association—click on "Healthcare Provider Directory")

To find an integrative physician (often experienced with fibro)
www.holisticmedicine.org (American Holistic Medical Association—click on "Find A Provider")
www.acam.org (American College for the Advancement of Medicine—click on "Health Resources" and then "Physician+Link")

2. Make 12 copies of and then complete the Personal Symptom Checklist (page 141) at the end of this chapter. You'll return to this worksheet in the coming weeks and months to record the status of your symptoms. Copy your completed list, date it, and give it to your doctor at your upcoming appointment, keeping the copy in your file.

3. Take the basal body temperature self-test for thyroid fatigue. Read "A do-it-yourself low-thyroid test: basal body temperature" (page 93), follow the instructions, and record your numbers. Clip them to a printed-out copy of the Physician's Guide to Fibromyalgia (page 299 + a printable PDF version at our website, wholehealthchicago.com) and hand it to your doctor at your appointment.

4. Ask your doctor to test your serotonin, norepinephrine, and adrenal gland function. Go to www.neurorelief.com

and click on "Patient Resources" and then "Refer your Doctor." Download the form, print, and in the space marked "Other" write "please order Test #9028 NeuroAdrenal Basic" and hand it to your doc. This test will measure your serotonin and norepinephrine levels and your adrenal gland function (read more about this neurotransmitter profile on page 85). It's covered by most health insurance companies. If your physician doesn't know about this lab, he or she will be grateful to learn about it. If your doctor says, "Don't bother me about this," say "thank you," leave, and return to Step 1 for help finding a physician who will be responsive.

5. Begin guided meditation. Go to Belleruth Naparstek's website Health Journeys (www.healthjourneys.com) and enter "fibromyalgia" into the search box. Then click on "Fibromyalgia & Chronic Fatigue" and purchase this guided meditation (you can download the MP3 to your iPod if you like). This totally wonderful healing meditation will help you release much of the fear you may have felt about your condition. Plan to listen at least three times a week. (Did you mark that on your calendar?)

6. Read the Fibro-Friendly Eating Plan (page 145) and start the Food Sensitivity Elimination-Reintroduction Eating Program. While you're paying attention to nutrition, begin eating primarily low-glycemic whole foods (fruits, vegetables, and protein) while eliminating white foods including white rice, white flour and everything made with it (pasta, bread, bakery goods), and sugar, including high-fructose corn syrup.

7. Begin gentle, daily exercise. Start by just walking—

around your neighborhood, outside during breaks at work, on an elliptical or treadmill, anything. Get in the sun for at least 30 minutes a day, using sunblock if needed but no sunglasses. Sunlight entering through your eyes kicks up your stress-protecting serotonin.

8. Locate a Myofascial Release Therapist and schedule a weekly visit. Go to www.myofascialrelease.com and click on "Find A Therapist." The select your state and see who's nearby. If resources are scant, search for a licensed massage therapist by the using the American Massage Therapy Association's therapist finder (www.amtamassage.org/-index.html). You're looking for a therapist who's familiar with fibromyalgia. Myofascial release is the ideal (but not the only) form of massage for fibro. For more on myofascial release, see Alternative Medicine for Fibromyalgia (page 245). Your physician can write you a prescription for myofascial release or massage therapy that may help with insurance reimbursement. If not, this therapy should be covered by your Health Savings Account if you have one.

9. Order these supplements and start taking them. They're all available online from many suppliers.

—**St. John's wort (SJW)** 450 mg twice daily (to raise your serotonin).
Don't take this without the supervision of a physician if you're already taking an SSRI antidepressant (though I use them together quite frequently in my practice as the SJW allows me to keep the SSRI dose low). Uncommon side effects of SJW include upset stomach, which you can avoid by taking with some food, and breakthrough bleeding if you're on a birth control pill.

—**Fish oil** 1000 mg (1 gram) two times daily, with meals. The omega-3 DHA (docosahexaenoic acid) in fish oil increases the amount of serotonin in your brain and enhances its efficiency. Krill oil, extracted from crustaceans, is a fine substitute.

—**B complex-100** One daily, with food.
Like fish oil, the B vitamins help your brain make more serotonin. They also help your liver flush out stress hormones, helping your nervous system stay on even keel.

—**5 Hydroxytryptophan (5HTP)** 100 mg at bedtime (to improve sleep and boost serotonin).
Like St. John's wort, 5HTP shouldn't be used with an SSRI without your physician's supervision. An uncommon side effect is next-day drowsiness. If this occurs, reduce your dose to 50 mg at bedtime.

—**Brain Energy (made by Douglas Labs)** Two capsules every morning.
This is a combination of two amino acids—D,L Phenylalanine and Tyrosine—that increase your brain level of norepinephrine with virtually no side effects.

By taking St. John's wort, 5HTP, and Brain Energy, you're essentially duplicating (but far more gently) the effects of Cymbalta and Savella, two FDA-approved prescription medications for fibromyalgia.

—**Fibroplex Plus** (made by Metagenics) One scoop twice daily.
This is a combination of magnesium, malic acid, and several vitamins. It's been clinically proven to reduce fibro pain and improve energy, and there are virtually no side effects.

—**AdrenPlus (made by Integrative Therapeutics)** Two capsules every morning.

This is a blend of herbs, vitamins, and amino acids for adrenal support. There are virtually no side effects.

—**Vitamin D** If your physician is willing to measure your vitamin D level and it is low, add supplemental vitamin D as needed. 2,000 IU (international units) daily is generally sufficient.

—**L-Theanine (made by Integrative Therapeutics)** If you're troubled by anxiety, take one capsule up to three times daily.

Ask Dr E: How Should I Prepare for My Doctor Visit?

With the introduction of FDA-approved medications for fibro, physician attitudes toward fibro are changing, and for the better. Nevertheless, I know of no condition that so demands that you be proactive in the healthcare system (I myself prefer "feisty" over "proactive") if you want to get well.

Here are some questions to bring to your physician, who may be your longstanding family doctor or someone new you've selected. Print out or copy this list and the Physician's Guide to Fibromyalgia (page 299 + a printable PDF version at our website, wholehealthchicago.com) and jot down the answers you receive.

The encounter can proceed as follows:

You (if you are undiagnosed): "I've been reading a lot about fibromyalgia in Dr Edelberg's book and I think this diagnosis explains a lot of my symptoms. I hurt everywhere, I'm tired all the time, and my tests have always been negative. He says the diagnosis can be confirmed by tender point examination. Would you please check mine?"

Your doctor (Answer #1): "There's no such thing as fibromyalgia. It's the latest fad diagnosis." If this occurs, thank the doctor, leave (mentally composing your blisteringly negative reviews on Yelp and Angie's List), and find a new doctor.

Your doctor (Answer #2): "Yes, fibromyalgia. We don't know much about it...There are some new medications...I'll refer you to a rheumatologist."

You (interrupting): "One moment, doctor. I've been doing a lot of reading about this and I really don't think I need to see a specialist. I have a short list of questions. Since this is a chronic condition, and I've been in pain for quite a while, your answers to these questions are important to me." Then hand your doctor this list and a pen:

—Have you prescribed any of the FDA-approved medications for fibro (Savella, Cymbalta, Lyrica)? Which do you prefer, and why?

—Would you be willing to prescribe these other medications for fibromyalgia:

- Muscle relaxants Y – N
- Pain medications (Tramadol, Vicodin, etc.) Y – N
- Sleep medications Y – N
- Energizers (Nuvigil, etc.) Y – N
- Antidepressants Y – N

—Would you write a prescription for physical therapy, myofascial release, or massage in an attempt to get my insurance to cover it? Y – N

—Would you read this Physician's Guide to Fibromyalgia (written by Dr Edelberg) that accompanied the book I've been reading? It's not long and contains no advertising. Y – N

—The Physician's Guide describes an easy-to-order test that measures neurotransmitter levels and adrenal function. After reading it, would you consider ordering that test? Y – N

—The book I'm reading recommends using nutritional supplements and alternative therapies like chiropractic, acupuncture, yoga, and stress reduction. Do you have a problem with any of these? Y – N

The purpose of having your physician answer these questions is not necessarily to guarantee a promise that he or she will actually do any of this. Rather, having read this list and holding a copy of the Physician's Guide, your doctor now has you firmly in mind as a proactive fibromyalgia patient, and this is extremely important as you move forward together.

Week 2: Writing Your Fibro Journal
(and a Good Hot Soak)

There is no "And on the seventh day, she rested" for you. We're moving right into Week 2, keeping in mind that these weekly guidelines are meant to be general. If it's happened to take you three weeks to arrive at this point, your attitude should be a nicely laid-back "Whatever..." Please don't get all tense about it. That's what we're trying to avoid.

If you've been working with the Week 1 tasks, at this point you should be:

- Scheduled with a physician (your usual doctor or a new one) to confirm your diagnosis and discuss your plans.

- Almost finished with this book.

- Seriously engaged in the Food Sensitivity Elimination-Reintroduction Eating Program (page 167).

- Looking at a completed Personal Symptoms Checklist (page 141).

- Doing something, *anything* for exercise every day: walking, treadmill, stationary bike, elliptical, hand weights, health club smorgasbord of various Inquisition-like devices (set the weight on "low").

- Going outside every day (sunlight, even through clouds,

will raise your serotonin).

- Having weekly myofascial release or massage.
- Listening to Belleruth Naparstek's Fibromyalgia & Chronic Fatigue guided meditation (details on page 108).
- Starting on the supplements listed in Week 1.

If you've not completed the Week 1 list, please do move forward with each step now.

On to Week 2, with just three tasks.

1. Write the story of your fibro in a journal. There is no medical condition for which the phrase "How your biography (your story) affects your biology" has more meaning than fibro. People with fibro always—always!—have a vital story to tell, and starting this week it's time to tell yours. If you haven't already read Memories in your Muscles (page 57), it's important to do so before you start journaling.

Get a bound notebook, open it to the first page and title it "The Story of My Fibro." Here are a few things to consider as you starting writing:

- **Look at the arc of your life, and the lives of your immediate biological family, for manifestations of low-serotonin stress susceptibility.** Did any of your relatives have depression, chronic anxiety, obsessive-compulsive symptoms, anger, or alcoholism/other drug dependence? They're all related to fibro's low-serotonin component and all part of the fibro spectrum (see The fibromyalgia spectrum on page 82). Equally important are family histories, especially those of your women relatives, because chronic fatigue, tension or migraine headaches, and irritable bowel syndrome are also related to low serotonin. One of my patients writing her journal wrote: "I remember mom saying every day how she hurt everywhere." That's a big clue—jot it down.

- **Review your own life, decade by decade, for memories of stressful events and physical symptoms.** Remember, fibromyalgia is all about stress. Were you the victim of bullying at school and as a result did you get such bad headaches or stomach aches on Monday mornings that you had to be kept home? Was there such chaos at home that you remember just sitting still, holding your body tight, waiting for the battles to end? Did you have an eating disorder as a teen? Ever relieve your anxiety with too much alcohol, marijuana, or other drugs? In your twenties, were you diagnosed with irritable bowel syndrome, depression, or anxiety? Include these snippets in your journal.

- **Now write about the year or two before the pain of fibromyalgia became a constant feature in your life.** Think about the stressors that triggered your fibro and the ones that are still around. You'd likely been carrying your stress in your neck and upper back for some reason. Did you start clenching your muscles after a rear-end whiplash auto accident, an interminable 90-minute commute, or a hellish job? Was it a divorce or a physical assault that preceded your fibro? Or another type of stress altogether—caring for a family member, trying to be a good mother while working two jobs, your financial situation disintegrating?

As you work on your journal and recognize the source of your fibromyalgia, you'll slowly feel your muscles begin to release themselves. Now you're understanding where your fibro came from, and also how stresses you currently face are keeping your fibro riled up.

We'll be working in Week 3 on naming and eliminating stress. If certain stressful aspects of your life simply cannot be changed ("My husband will always be my husband. I can't leave."), consider professional counseling to learn some coping strategies other than painfully locking up your muscles.

For more on all this, take a look at Mary's Fibro Journal on page 117 just below to see how she recorded the threads that make up the tapestry of her fibro story.

If you're suffering from depression or chronic anxiety, two of the most common low-serotonin mood disorders, consider scheduling an appointment with a psychologist along with your journaling efforts. Working with a therapist becomes especially important if you can trace your fibromyalgia to unresolved emotionally traumatic events that you've not come to terms with, like an abusive childhood, a marriage from hell, or the loss of a loved one.

Keep in mind, though, that a majority of fibro patients who have been incorrectly diagnosed as "depressed" are experiencing a perfectly normal emotional response to the constant pain and perpetual exhaustion. If you're one of the many whose symptoms have not been taken seriously, and you see no bright star on the horizon, you probably don't need psychotherapy: you simply need to feel better. Writing down your story and following all the steps in this plan will help.

Patient Stories: Mary's Fibro Journal

Here are some sentences from Mary's fibro journal. She's still indecisive about sharing it with her husband, Dean, as he's "tired of me being tired and might not understand how all this relates to that."

"I am 42 years old, married, with two wonderful teenagers, and as I sit here writing this I realize that I've been in pain for five straight years."

"I think that as a child my family meant well. I know my parents loved me, but they had serious problems of their own. I've often wondered if they would have been happier if they'd never married (there was that much fighting)."

"Dad came from an abusive home himself, so I've always cut him a lot of slack even though he could be horrible at times. He had a real problem with alcohol and anger. I've never even told Dean about it. I remember being so scared as a kid."

"Today, mom would be diagnosed with depression, but being Scandinavian, she kept everything to herself. Her doctor once recommended Prozac, but she refused to consider it."

"My oldest sister has panic attacks and my brother drinks far too much and smokes a lot of pot."

"My parents finally got divorced when I was ten. We had to move a lot because there was no money. I hated going to school because my clothes were secondhand. I had a lot of stomach aches."

"I don't remember ever being happy in high school. I got good grades, but always felt like an outsider. I used to get these stress headaches and my neck was always sore. I was an overachiever and I can see now I was trying to compensate for what was going on at home."

"In college, I remember having terrible diarrhea around finals, all the stress triggering what was probably irritable bowel syndrome. When I think it about now, I think I drank too much to try to ease the stress."

"I was healthy in my twenties, but I broke up with Bob after three years of promises and an abortion, and then I was really depressed. I took Zoloft and it helped, but I gained 20 pounds and I've never been able to lose it."

"The babies came after I married Dean. I had some postpartum depression, but otherwise everything seemed fine until Dean lost his job and our house went into foreclosure. Then mom got really sick and needed me every day and the stress was intense. I started feeling like I was crumbling, so tired and so stressed. I think that's when my fibro began."

Mary's fibro story runs to eight neatly written pages. Her final sentence: "I think I can see how this all started and I feel better just writing it down."

2. Begin taking a nightly hot soak in the bathtub. You'll need this quiet time to think (and maybe cry a little) about your journal entries. Fill your tub with very warm water, adding a cup of Epsom salts and a few drops of lavender oil. Ask anyone you live with to leave you alone for an hour.

Light a candle, turn off the overhead light, play some relaxing music, lie back quietly, and allow your muscles to open themselves. Release the story of your fibro, forgiving those who caused you pain and locked up your muscles. Let go of the stress that's accumulated over this life. Open your mind to feeling good again, knowing you have this book as a guide.

3. Assuming you've seen your (usual or new) doctor once, schedule a return visit ten days or two weeks from now. It's an important step we'll cover in Week 4.

Week 3: Introduce potential food culprits, document stress reduction, boost exercise, and eat green and orange

You're now into your second or third week of both the supplements and the Food Sensitivity Elimination-Reintroduction Eating Program (page 167). You've experienced at least one weekly session of myofascial release therapy (or a decent massage) and you've discussed your plans with your doctor. You're relaxing in a nightly hot bath, regularly listening to Belleruth Naparstek's Fibromyalgia & Chronic Fatigue guided meditation (page 108), and journaling the story of your fibro, listing the different manifestations of your low-serotonin stress susceptibility. You're starting to see when your fibro first began.

1. Start reintroducing potential food culprits (details on page 167). I'll admit when you begin many different therapies simultaneously and then start to feel better it's difficult to determine what's working. The answer is *everything*. Every step you take — from reading this book to cleaning up your diet, from acknowledging your stressors to going for a walk — is helping. If there were a single magic-bullet fibro cure I would have shared it on page 1.

I do believe that in about a third of people with fibro, food sensitivities (not allergies, but sensitivities) contribute to the stress that triggers the muscle contractions of fibro. Doctors who work in the field of nutritional medicine, and clinical nutritionists themselves, have heard the phrase "I feel so much better since I stopped eating gluten (or dairy or whatever)!" too often to chalk it up to coincidence.

Certain foods are simply toxic to susceptible individuals, usually women with low-serotonin sensitivities, which also manifest as sensitivities to prescription drugs, the weather, scents, and chemicals.

Before your start the reintroduction, make sure you've been off the following foods for at least two weeks (maybe longer, that's fine): dairy, egg, corn, citrus, soy, and gluten grains. Then begin reintroducing one food group at a time. Of the six, the most common culprit is wheat (and other gluten grains) so save its reintroduction for last.

As you begin returning one food group to your diet every three days, make notes in your journal. As you introduce a food, *pay careful attention to how you feel, physically and emotionally.*

Common symptoms of a hidden food sensitivity include:

- muscle and joint aching
- fatigue
- headache
- digestive symptoms (heartburn, gas, nausea, bloating)
- sinus congestion
- skin breakouts
- moodiness
- depression

If you experience any of these during the three-day reintroduction of a food group, stop eating that food altogether (again) and move on to the next food group to reintroduce. If after a full three days of eating the reintroduced food group you feel fine, you can continue eating it and move on to reintroducing the next one.

Ultimately, you'll be eating only those foods welcomed by your body, that "welcome" being expressed by the complete absence of any unpleasant symptoms.

2. Itemize the steps you'll take toward stress reduction. It's back to your fibro journal again, in a section separate from the story of your fibro. Title it STRESS REDUCTION and begin by learning the pronunciation of "No," as in "No, I'm so sorry I can't be a part of that." Devote a whole page to the word NO, written in large block letters (so that you remember both the pronunciation and the spelling). Decorate that page with a lot of little "no's." Refer to it often.

Your "No" page applies to all aspects of your life—family, work, and personal relationships. Write down what stresses you out. Think about the changes you need to make in your life, like resigning from that committee you're sorry you joined, asking your siblings to help with the care of your parents, or stopping the volunteer work at your child's school ("It's just temporary," you can say, "until I'm feeling more energetic."). If they keep pushing, say "I'm so sorry I can't right now—doctor's orders."

Cut back on all unnecessary obligations, social events, and extra projects at work if possible. Do not, under any circumstances, start any project that might increase stress.

Think about which parts of your life require minimal stress for maximum return. Do you relax when you have friends over for dinner or is a one huge stress-provoking event? Could the format be changed to a potluck, where everyone contributes a dish? Perhaps you'll choose to meet those same friends outside your home, requiring minimal work by you. Or invite people who make you feel relaxed to your home for a cup of tea.

Or...and I know this sounds drastic...take a break altogether from socializing. Remember, "I'm so sorry I can't right now — doctor's orders."

Expand your stress reduction possibilities. Could you say no to your commute by finding a job closer to home? Consider that it's entirely possible for your teenagers to do their own laundry and teach them how. It's a valuable life skill, just as helping with dinner and clean-up are.

Go slowly with your list, remembering you need to learn to crawl before you walk. Make two categories: "stress reduction I can do now" and "ideas to work on."

3. Ramp up exercise a bit. Yes, I'm impressed you've been walking more, on the elliptical or simply outside. Now, turn up the resistance on the machine or add some one or two-pound hand/leg weights during your outdoor walk.

Walk farther and, oh yes, a little faster. Examine your day and imagine how you might increase activity, such as walking to the grocery store, parking farther from the mall entrance, or leaving public transport two stops early and hiking the difference to your workplace.

Do you spend Sunday mornings in a prone position with coffee and the news, the internet, or a movie? Switch it up, even briefly. Get up, throw on some comfy clothes, drink a large glass of water, eat a piece of fruit and a hard-boiled egg, and walk outside — however far you can. Take time to relax later in the day.

4. Increase your consumption of green and orange veggies. Your body is extraordinarily adept at extracting the vitamins, minerals, and antioxidants it needs from food rather than pills. Supplements can be helpful, but your body is hard-wired to know healthy food when you eat it. Honor this knowledge and your body will reward you with steadily increasingly good health.

Return to the Fibro-Friendly Eating Plan (page 145) this week to reacquaint yourself with good nutrition principles and foods that boost serotonin while preventing adrenal fatigue and low blood sugar, both of which exacerbate fibro by placing even more stress on your body.

As part of all this, increase your intake green and orange vegetables: cabbage (make slaw); deep green lettuces, spinach, and other greens (make salads); and broccoli, peas, green beans, and asparagus (steam and add olive oil). Cut up brightly colored raw veggies like carrots and summer squash (zucchini and yellow squash) to eat mid-afternoon. Cook sweet potatoes year-round (dice them and they'll steam in 20 minutes) and make pumpkin and winter squash a permanent menu feature in the winter months.

Fibro Quicksand: Not staying active

Virtually every study shows that regular exercise is extremely effective in reducing fibro symptoms. But because of pain and fatigue, women with fibro can easily turn into chronically inactive couch potatoes. In the process, many (in fact, most) become overweight.

If this is you, read the Fibro-Friendly Eating Plan (page 145) for ideas on how to clean up your diet and use food as a tool in treating your fibro.

But back to being active. This doesn't mean you start training for a triathlon tomorrow, OK? Begin by walking every day, lengthening the time and distance and picking up speed over a period of weeks. As your energy strengthens, gradually diversify and intensify.

Walk the stairs, get outside at lunch, stretch. Just keep moving, remembering to take frequent breaks. One of my patients, Phyllis, started a stair-walking group at work. At 3 pm every day (when most of her colleagues are hitting the vending machines) Phyllis's small band of stair-walkers get going. When they're finished, they head for their water bottles, apple, and cheese.

Try it. Even if you can manage just one flight to start, you'll be astounded at the ability of your body to adapt and you'll be walking higher every week.

If you're at home, start by walking your neighborhood and doing some light chores every day (but please share the hard ones with other family members). Take stairs whenever possible, park at the far end of the lot and walk the maximum distance, do some gardening—all the usual advice to fit in activity whenever possible.

As your strength increases, sample yoga, Pilates, biking, exercise tapes, swimming, weights (light ones to start, please), or home exercise equipment. If money's no object, hire a personal trainer for a couple hours to teach you some basic strengthening moves you can do at home. Or sign up for a health club membership.

It almost goes without saying: Spend less time on the internet and in front of your TV and more time moving.

Week 4: Your Return Visit to the Doctor

Seeing your doctor for a follow-up visit is your only task for Week 4. It's that important. But you have a little homework to do before leaving home. Read through this entire week's assignment and develop the presentation I'm suggesting so it's complete…before you go. In preparation, update a copy of the Personal Symptom Checklist (page 141) and date it. Make two copies of everything: one for you and one for your doc.

Maintain your routine of healthy eating and culprit food reintroduction, supplements, guided meditation, gradually increasing exercise, sun exposure, journaling, stress reduction, and weekly myofascial release or massage.

You might also make a journal entry on your feelings about your visit with the doctor.

1. Make the return visit to your physician. With luck, she's glanced through the Physician's Guide to Fibromyalgia so the two of you can talk together about next steps. If she's managed to lose it (doctors get flooded with paper), she can find a printable PDF version at our website, wholehealthchicago.com.

Remembering that all primary care doctors are overworked and spend less time with patients than they'd like, it's your job as a proactive fibro patient to make your office visit as efficient as possible. Believe me, your doctor will appreciate your organization.

Begin with a variation of: Hi, remember me? I'm your proactive fibro patient on a six-week plan. By the way, did you get a chance to read Dr Edelberg's Physician's Guide to Fibro I gave you last time?

Then follow these steps:

- Present an organized list of the supplements you've been taking from Week 1. Unless your doctor has read the Physician's Guide or has a special interest in nutritional medicine, she's going to look blankly at some of the items on your list. She'll know B complex and fish oil, but may draw a blank on St. John's Wort and 5HTP. Quickly educate her: "The St John's and 5HTP raise my serotonin. The Brain Energy boosts my norepinephrine. Same mechanism as Cymbalta and Savella." Don't digress. Don't get humble and ask, "Is it all right to take these?" If she doesn't know what they're for, she'll say no.

- Present a second organized list of everything you're doing. Describe your eating program, increased physical activity, bodywork therapies (massage), and stress reduction. Believe me, at this point you're piquing the doctor's interest. She will visibly appear less harried and more focused on you. She's thinking, "If this patient is feeling better, it's something I can offer my other fibro patients. Where did I put that Physician's Guide?"

- Present your updated Personal Symptom Checklist for comparison with the original. Be sure it's dated and let your doctor know it's an extra copy for your office chart.

- If during Week 1 you submitted a NeuroScience test kit for neurotransmitter and adrenal function, ask if the results are back from the lab. Remember that this test is likely going to be new to your doctor, so she may be hesitant about interpreting the results. You'll mainly be looking at serotonin levels (generally low), norepinephrine levels (also low), cortisol levels from your adrenal gland (also low), and DHEA (also adrenal gland-related and also low). You are in the process of raising serotonin with the St. John's wort, fish oil, and 5HTP; the norepinephrine with Brain Energy; and adrenal function with AdrenPlus. If your cortisol level is extremely low, your doctor may want to give you a small dose of prescription cortisol (called Cortef). If all your tests are either normal or better than expected, this does not change your fibromyalgia diagnosis or the steps you've been following in this chapter. The NeuroScience test gives a useful overview, but it does not diagnose the condition. There are no diagnostic tests for fibro. Period.

- Present her with the results of your basal body temperature thyroid test. If your temperatures are low (below 97.6), ask if she would write a prescription for a small (30-mg) dose of Armour thyroid. She may prefer synthetic Synthroid (Levoxyl) at 50 mcg instead. That's an acceptable second choice. It's not worth arguing about as the time allotted for your appointment is likely quite short.

- Now the most challenging part. With all the paperwork delivered, you need to face the reality of how you think you're doing with your fibro so far. Although improvement after four weeks is more apparent for some patients than others, I've never seen anyone get worse. Likely, you'll say one of three things:

1. "I really think I'm doing better and I'm going to continue down this path. No prescriptions (except for the thyroid medication and maybe something for my adrenal glands when that test comes back)."

2. "I'm not worse, but I'm not much better either. I'd like to talk about prescription medications. Maybe one of the three FDA-approved drugs for fibro, or at least something for pain, like time-release tramadol." Note: if you start either Savella or Cymbalta, you'll discontinue St. John's wort, 5HTP, and Brain Energy.

3. "I have a very specific symptom that this program isn't addressing. Is there anything you can give me to help with...(sleep, energy, mood, restless legs, etc.)

- Ask for the prescriptions you need for medications, physical therapy, myofascial release/massage therapy. Don't be shy: you'll use these prescriptions to get

127

insurance reimbursement for your out-of-pocket expenses.

• Schedule a follow-up visit in about one month.

Week 5: Yoga

If you've been diligent about following this plan, your body is slowly adjusting to the changes you've made. What seemed like a large number of pills to be swallowing twice daily is now second nature and really, by this time, you may be feeling the serotonin/norepinephrine boost of St. John's wort and Brain Energy and the muscle- relaxing effects of magnesium in the Fibroplex Plus.

Large parts of your self-care routine are becoming habit—well done. You're certainly more physically active than you were a month ago. People around you are aware that you're on a path to wellness. Your family notices healthier food served at meals (as does your body), and your "I'm going out for my walk" is by now familiar to them. Everyone knows the bathtub is yours for a certain hour each evening.

1. This week, begin yoga, both for your fibro and to reduce stress, though I'll admit the two are inseparable.

Clinical studies from around the world have shown that regardless of age, people who practice yoga are healthier than the rest of the population. They're more relaxed and have more energy, better strength and joint flexibility, lower blood pressure, slower pulses, stronger hearts, better sleep, improved digestion, and more positive outlooks on life.

In fact, starting regular yoga practice this week will allow you to finally walk away from the pain and fatigue of fibro.

Emotionally, yoga students have increased self-awareness,

better coping skills, and a more relaxed approach to any stress, whether job-related or caused by family crisis. This may be partially due to the slew of feel-good endorphins released during yoga postures. Among these endorphins are serotonin and norepinephrine, the same two you've been boosting with your supplement regimen. It's also the same pair targeted by the fibro meds Savella and Cymbalta.

Doctors like me who practice integrative medicine regularly recommend yoga classes as complementary therapy for such conditions as fibro, chronic fatigue, migraine, irritable bowel syndrome, depression, panic and anxiety disorders, arthritis, and even cancer. It's just fine during pregnancy, too, and many hospitals now offer prenatal yoga classes.

Start with a class

Without a doubt, in-person yoga classes are superior to videotape instruction. And, honestly, you need to live in a pretty remote area of the US to be unserved by yoga classes somewhere nearby. Why an actual class? You need a little guidance as you first learn the postures, and then you'll be able to move along at your own pace. Remember that yoga instructors are not health care professionals and as such no formal licensing is required. It's probably a good idea to ask about your instructor's training, certification, and the number of years she's been teaching. In addition, tell him or her about any health issues that might require some adjustment to your individual routine, including your (ever-improving) fibro.

Some people prefer a morning session to energize them throughout the day. Others choose an evening class to move them into deep sleep. Whatever time you select, arrive with an empty stomach and don't plan to eat for at least an hour afterward. All classes come to a close with a few minutes of deep relaxation, a roomful of students sprawled comfortably and blissfully across the floor. Fibro patients tell me they can actually feel the knots in their muscles open up and the blood coursing through them, washing away accumulated toxins.

Plan to schedule one or, even better, two yoga sessions a week, during which you'll also learn techniques for daily practice. Yoga classes are usually about an hour long, and your daily at-home practice can be 20 to 30 minutes. If you're uncertain which form of yoga is right for you, try a few and see which is most appealing. Bear in mind that you'll be more inclined to stick with a class that's geographically convenient and fits into your schedule.

And like everything else in life, attending class regularly for about three weeks makes it a habit, and a good one at that. The integration of mind and body will allow you to feel a real sense of calm and peacefulness. Stress will melt away as you feel yourself becoming centered. As muscle tension disappears, every joint feels more limber and flexible.

A word about Bikram Yoga

Although the idea of doing yoga postures in a room heated to 105 degrees may sound daunting, if you've got a Bikram center in your area, I'd recommend you give it a try.

Despite the heat, the Bikram postures are actually easier to perform than other forms of yoga, probably because the external heat is doing most of the work for you. The classes are 90 minutes long and during that period you'll assume 26 postures (each is performed twice) plus two breathing exercises.

If you're unfamiliar with either the Bikram method or yoga in any form, I suggest meeting with the school's director, explaining your fibro and asking for a shorter private session or two that covers some of the easier postures, so you can starting training yourself to reach the full 90 minutes.

Why Bikram is so helpful is simple enough. Every person with fibro knows she's in less pain when her muscles are warm and in more pain when she's cold. It makes little difference whether that warmth comes from a hot tub or shower, a summer day, or a baking beach in Puerto Vallarta. Warm is better. To be able to stretch those knotted fibro muscles when every one of them has been heated becomes the ideal self-treatment.

Over the years, dozens of fibro patients have related to me how yoga practice, whether in class or using a DVD at home, helped pain, flexibility, energy, and stress. When the Bikram studios began opening around Chicago and my patients experimented with what seemed like the latest fad from California, the results were remarkable.

Week 6: Structuring A Life Without Fibro

By following this plan so far, you've integrated healthy eating, regular exercise, guided meditation, and yoga into your life. Did you realize when we began how essential they'd be to overcoming your fibro?

The nutritional supplements from Week 1 are having a real impact on how you feel. And you've located a sympathetic, fibro-educated physician who's supporting your considerable efforts. You've made enormous strides.

Every evening you're soaking in a hot bath, visualizing your muscles releasing their painful knots and opening up. You're pleased with the decisions you've made so far to eliminate busy-ness activities and reduce stress. You may understand you have more to do, but you know you're getting well and because of your journaling you now "get" how fibro got you.

So what's this about structuring a life without fibro? Isn't that what you've been doing? Absolutely. But there's some fine-tuning to be done in order to craft a schedule—a life, really—that keeps the chaff off your plate and leaves spaces for what's needed to feel even better and stay well.

The most important thought you can have right now: I'm never returning to Fibro Land. Wait, you might say, I'm feeling better. How could that happen? How could my fibromyalgia come back? All too easily, I'm afraid. Many of my fibromyalgia patients making progress with this six-week program have a tendency to start doing too much once they're feeling better, returning to the days of packing in activities and obligations, exercising too hard, or forgetting about their yoga and guided meditation.

I salute your efforts to pull yourself out of fibro's grip, but understand your muscles are still susceptible to soreness and your energy reserves aren't yet up to snuff. Take it slowly to avoid rebounding and feeling discouraged.

Maintaining a fibro-free life takes consistent planning and organization

First, check to see that you've covered everything in this chapter. Refer to your fibro journal to ensure you have:

- Kept current with the food sensitivity elimination-reintroduction plan as well as the larger eating program.

- Maintained your daily supplement regimen.

- Done your twice-weekly guided meditation.

- Walked daily, and steadily increased your activity.

- Scheduled your weekly myofascial release massage.

- Stretched through your yoga positions.

- Carefully re-examined (again!) your life for stressors and taken steps to eliminate them.

- Cried, and cried some more, about the triggers that brought fibro to your doorstep and then realized you could walk away from it all and be the pain-free, vital, and active woman you were meant to be.

But, you might be thinking, I really am trying to do it all but I'm just *too busy* to go to a yoga class and certainly can't find a quiet spot for meditating in this house.

I'll be the first to admit this nearly natural cure relies mostly on you. It's not as easy as swallowing your daily supplements, though that's certainly a part of it. Your assiduous attention to detail this week—and every week of your future—is your insurance against a return of the worst manifestations of fibromyalgia.

Even if you're in charge of a family and also hold a paying job (many of my patients do both), you need to think about structuring a life that gives you time to:

Honor the progress you've made with the fibro-friendly eating approach. Step it up, even. Are you making and taking your lunch and snacks to work? Planning time on the weekend to cook healthful foods and freezing for the week ahead? Or have you slipped back into the old habit of grabbing a bag of chips during your afternoon slump, eating whatever swill they're serving in the cafeteria for lunch, and turning to frozen pizza for dinner? Reinvigorate your efforts with the food plan (page 145), bringing family members into the shopping and preparing. You're all going to feel a lot healthier for it.

Nurture yourself. You're physically and emotionally more sensitive than people who don't have fibro (not necessarily a bad thing). Respect that sensitivity by not overdoing it. Going back to a life of endless racing around, overscheduling, and not planning time for the healing activities in this chapter is a GPS route directly to Fibro Land.

Schedule essential tasks, including re-ordering the supplements that are keeping you strong. You might laugh at this one, but we all have our to-do lists and maintaining your supply of the supplements listed in Week 1 can easily fall off your radar. Think of it as keeping your life-support line plugged in, right along with showing up for yoga and myofascial or other massage. I'll admit it's easier—and sometime seems like more fun—to throw down in front of the TV or go out with friends. Take the time now to schedule essential tasks just as you'd schedule something for your daughter's birthday.

Eliminate the unnecessarily stressful parts of your life. I can't say it often enough. Return to your journal page titled Stress Reduction and give it an honest review. Have you cut back on social obligations that generate more stress than stress-free enjoyment? Learned to say "no"? Looked clearly at how you spend time doing tasks that have to be done (laundry, food shopping) and structured your time to release the pressure? Organizing beats haphazard every time.

Two examples: Camille and Grace

Let's look at the different approaches taken by two of my patients as a way to illustrate all this. You may fall somewhere between the two, but there are lessons to be learned from both.

First, Camille, who worked through the nearly natural cure like she did everything—with careful attention to detail. She took each step seriously, located a smart and sympathetic new physician, had some eye-opening epiphanies while writing her journal, and was as ruthless as anyone I've treated about cutting back on stress.

This is what she told me one day, with a laugh, a few months into her efforts.

"Sometimes I feel my life is like my grandmother's. She's 90 and lives in a care facility where all meals and activities are rigidly scheduled. But you know what I realized just this week? I feel 100% better when I don't over-schedule or overdo. I feel better physically *and* mentally when I take time for my healthy breakfast before I leave the house and my fast walking during lunch hour, when I get home with enough time to enjoy making a real meal with my boys.

"My weekly yoga class is sacrosanct, and my husband knows it's his night to help the kids with homework and do mid-week laundry. I finally figured out I could tolerate one social outing per week...and I save it for the weekend."

Camille, still young at 38, had made a real effort to organize her life in a fibro-calming way. She was shopping on the weekends and cooking big batches of real food, assisted by her two children, enjoying the process and saving money to boot.

"My kids actually now say 'Hey, maybe we can have that chili tonight for supper.' They're actually getting good at food prep."

Camille held a high-profile, high-stress position at a management company and quickly saw she needed to reserve a lot of her energy to keep up with it.

"Yes, there are still days my boss is demanding beyond belief, but I find I roll with those days better when I live a structured life the rest of the time. Kind of like my grandma."

Camille still has some loose ends. She's in therapy (working on resolving what her mother put her through as a child), and still has some weight to lose, but she's developing a plan for that too. Overall, though, Camille is engaged and in charge of her fibro.

And now Grace, whose first visit began with this challenge, "You're the twentieth doctor I've seen. They say I have fibromyalgia, but I don't know. I don't think anyone can help me."

She'd handed me a shopping bag full of medical records. I reviewed them and quickly confirmed her diagnosis before we discussed fibro at length. Then I gave her some material I'd written and placed her on the six-week plan you've so assiduously completed.

Six weeks later, Grace was back and definitely not smiling.

Here's our exchange:

Me: So, are you making any progress?

Grace: None at all. I'm exactly the same. In fact, I think I'm worse. My pain is worse and I'm so tired I can barely move. I was thinking about cancelling this appointment, but wanted to know my test results.

We reviewed these together, with me relaying that, indeed, her serotonin and norepinephrine were low. Also, her adrenal glands were exhausted. I asked Grace if she'd taken her basal body temperature and she told me she hadn't had time to do it.

Me: Right, so how are you doing with the supplements?

Grace: I had some other vitamins at home so I didn't buy any new ones. Yours looked more expensive than Walmart and I figured I didn't really need more.

Me: Have you tried the myofascial release therapy?

Grace: My insurance wouldn't cover it.

Me: Did you begin the detox eating program? (I didn't really have to bother asking…)

Now, you might reasonably ask, "What's going on here? Why is Grace suffering so needlessly and seeing so many doctors, but not following any advice or instructions?"

And my answer would be that people are far more complicated than they appear. Being a physician is more than listening to patients relate their symptoms and writing prescriptions. Most of us (doctors and patients alike) think everyone should be motivated to get well, but sadly this is not the case.

Likely Grace herself is completely unaware of the

unconscious reasons for what psychologists would call her resistance to feeling better.

In her particular case, she was an attorney in a brutally stressful practice and at one point told me she'd never wanted to be a lawyer in the first place (she took that path thinking it would make her father happy). Some time after she developed fibro, she took a six-week medical leave and felt better after two weeks. As it came time for her to return to work, her fibro worsened (my smart readers know why: stress). Grace is now on disability and too ill to consider returning to work.

The one thing she did remember during our visit was to bring the forms for me to complete to extend her disability coverage.

Is Grace a hopeless case? Is this her life, constantly struggling with pain and fatigue, dragging behind her an ever-expanding suitcase of medical records, travelling from doctor to doctor?

Not hopeless, but definitely the antithesis of Camille. What's needed is for Grace to work with a skilled and compassionate clinical psychologist who can explore with her the reasons for her fibromyalgia and give her "permission" to make the life changes that would help her out of this rut.

What To Do If the Nearly Natural Approach Isn't Working

Even with devoted effort to the six-week plan, some people with more intractable fibro need extra help. Don't feel discouraged. Your next steps are right here:

1. Learn how the FDA-approved fibro drugs work in the small doses I recommend Read Medications for Fibro: How They Work and How They Can Help (page 187) to understand how my dosing schedule for Savella, Cymbalta, or Lyrica can help your fibro while limiting medication side effects.

2. Hand your doctor the Physician's Guide (page 299 + a printable PDF version at our website, wholehealthchicago.com) and ask him or her to help you get started on a low dose of one of the FDA-approved fibro drugs. They can take up to six weeks to ramp up and take effect.

The two FDA-approved medications that correct fibro's fundamental abnormalities (low serotonin and low norepinephrine) are Savella and Cymbalta. To avoid side effects, ask your doctor to write their prescriptions following my dosing schedule in the Physician's Guide. If you begin either of these medications, stop taking the St. John's wort, 5HTP, and DLPA/Tyrosine. The fibro meds do the same thing as the supplements, but are more potent.

Lyrica, the third FDA-approved fibro medication, can be an effective pain medication and can be used in combination with supplements. Watch your weight carefully if you chose Lyrica, since weight gain can occur if you're not paying attention.

3. Review the section "Other helpful fibro medicines" on page 212 and use your intuition to sense which ones might be helpful for issues you haven't been able to resolve with the Nearly Natural Cure.

Then discuss these other medicines with your doctor. He or

she will find information on them in the Physician's Guide (page 299 + a printable PDF version at our website, wholehealthchicago.com):

- Pain medication (tramadol, hydrocodone, oxycodone)
- Sleep medication (Ambien, Lunesta, Trazodone)
- Muscle relaxants (Flexeril, Amrix — time release Flexeril)
- Energizers (Provigil, Nuvigil)
- Antidepressants

Starting prescription medication simply means you'll be taking fewer supplements. The rest of your fibromyalgia program remains in place.

This means continuing myofascial massage, journaling, increased physical activity, healthful eating, guided meditation, and stress reduction. These are essential components to putting your fibromyalgia behind you.

Personal Symptom Checklist
Date_____

Tracking your fibro is essential, and that's how you'll use this form. Right upfront, print out or copy a dozen clean copies. You'll use them to track your symptoms over time and you'll also bring a completed checklist to every visit with your physician (keeping a copy of the completed form for your files).

Fibro's hallmark symptoms are muscle pain and fatigue, the first two on this checklist. Grade their status from 1 to 10, with 10 being most severe.

Fibromyalgia spectrum symptoms make up the rest of the checklist. People with fibro suffer a range of these symptoms, all caused by a low level of stress-buffering serotonin, which causes your fight-or-flight stress response (for emergency use only) to be activated almost constantly. Rate the fibro spectrum symptoms from 1 to 5, with 5 being most severe.

Complete the questionnaire now, date it, and place it in a folder marked Fixing My Fibro. You'll be completing this again a month from now, and every month thereafter.

Muscle pain
(least) 1 2 3 4 5 6 7 8 9 10 (most)

Fatigue
(least) 1 2 3 4 5 6 7 8 9 10 (most)

Stiffness (on waking up or after prolonged sitting)
(least) 1 2 3 4 5 (most) **or N/A** (not applicable/never a problem)

Brain fog (poor focus, memory issues)
(least) 1 2 3 4 5 (most) **or N/A**

Headache (tension or migraine)
(least) 1 2 3 4 5 (most) **or N/A**

TMJ (jaw clenching/grinding)
(least)1 2 3 4 5 (most) **or N/A**

Sleep disturbances
(least) 1 2 3 4 5 (most) **or N/A**

Unrefreshing sleep
(least) 1 2 3 4 5 (most) **or N/A**

Sensation of skin/muscle swelling
(least) 1 2 3 4 5 (most) **or N/A**

Pelvic pain (including any previous diagnosis of interstitial cystitis)
(least) 1 2 3 4 5 (most) **or N/A**

Painful intercourse
(least) 1 2 3 4 5 (most) **or N/A**

Multiple chemical sensitivities (you get side effects from most drugs, perfumes and other chemical smells make you feel sick, etc)
(least) 1 2 3 4 5 (most) **or N/A**

Depression
(least) 1 2 3 4 5 (most) or **N/A**

Symptoms worse in winter
(least) 1 2 3 4 5 (most) or **N/A**

Symptoms affected by weather
(least) 1 2 3 4 5 (most) **or N/A**

Symptoms worse during PMS days or when menopause started
(least) 1 2 3 4 5 (most) or **N/A**

Irritable bowel syndrome (bloating, nausea, diarrhea, constipation, abdominal cramps)
(least) 1 2 3 4 5 (most) **or N/A**

Poor sense of overall well-being
(least) 1 2 3 4 5 (most) **or N/A**

9

FIBRO-FRIENDLY EATING PLAN

You'll notice, I hope, that this isn't called a fibro diet. I assiduously avoid the D word because it implies a lack of permanence, as in "I won't have to do *this* forever." You know how it goes: you resolve to start a new diet with a lurking agenda in the back of your mind that on some glorious day when you've reached your goal you can go off the diet and eat "normally" again.

Let's face it. The "some glorious day" approach is seriously unrealistic, whether you're eating to permanently keep weight off or keep your fibromyalgia under control. This eating plan is, yes indeed-y, a "rest of your life" undertaking. Honestly, once you start eating primarily real foods and feel so-o-o-o much better, you won't crave junk food, sugar, and other fast carbs the way you probably do now.

Indeed, rest-of-your-life eating would sound ominous were it not for some significantly pleasant and motivating perks. In addition to feeling less physical discomfort from your fibro and having more energy, on this eating plan, you will:

- Live longer.
- Lose weight, especially once you master the art of portion control.
- Reduce your risk of developing heart disease, diabetes,

and some cancers.

After decades of being a doctor, I can safely say that most people, especially when they're traipsing through the foothills of middle age, if offered a choice between the Biblical three score and ten and the 21st century's four score and ten select the path with the extra two decades.

The Fibro-Friendly Eating Plan includes several strategies directed toward your uniqueness as a person with fibromyalgia. As you're well aware by now, fibromyalgia primarily affects women with low levels of the stress-buffering neurotransmitter serotonin. That means you, more than others, are vulnerable to stress in any form. **Common sense then tells us that healthful fibro eating has two basic principles: raising serotonin and lowering stress.**

This chapter discusses a variety of strategies to achieve just that. Now you might say, "I can understand there might be foods that raise my serotonin. I've read about those. But how can food lower stress unless I'm swallowing a Valium before dinner?"

The answer is that certain seemingly innocuous foods might be very stressful to your body, ultimately exhausting your adrenal glands. When you're sensitive to foods, every time you eat them your body experiences a low-level but predictable fight-or-flight response. Subject your adrenal glands to hourly fight-or-flight and you can expect adrenal fatigue.

Like many fibromyalgia patients, you may also be highly chemically sensitive. When you eat processed foods, laced with the finest pesticides, herbicides, and preservatives science has to offer, your body may respond with the same horror and shock as if you were sipping toxic dump run-off.

Devour chemical swill and expect adrenal fatigue.

And again like many fibro patients, you may be exquisitely sensitive to abrupt shifts in blood sugar levels, experiencing the predictable fight-or-flight response whenever you're hypoglycemic (have low blood sugar). Addicted to sugar-y, fast-carb foods, expect adrenal fatigue.

Therefore, eating to reduce stress means eliminating:

- Foods you're sensitive to.
- Foods containing chemicals, additives, or preservatives.
- Foods that can trigger periods of hypoglycemia.

I promise this isn't a difficult plan to follow. You'll undoubtedly be saying a fond farewell to a lot of childhood favorites, like Twinkies, Little Debbies, and Count Chocula. You'll never under any circumstances (except perhaps to use their restroom) cross the threshold of any fast-food restaurant ever again.

Don't be daunted by all the sections. The reason I've separated them is so you'll clearly understand why you'll be eating more of one type of food and less of (or even eliminating) another. You need to have your own personal "Aha!" moment when you make the connection between food and fibro.

Read through this chapter once and you'll quickly see how the pieces fit together...and how returning to a diet of real foods is central to all aspects of the plan.

Patient Stories: Eve Makes the Connection
Between Food and Fibro

It's true that the vast majority of people with fibro eat poorly and it's well-established that a majority are overweight.

A new patient I'll call Eve was no exception. She'd struggled for years with her weight and her fibro and, like most fibro patients who come to our clinic, she didn't see any connection between how she was feeling (pain, fatigue, weakness) and the nutritional content of her diet. Eve's pantry and fridge held a wealth of sugar-free, carb-reduced "diet" foods that contained lots of chemical additives and imitation flavors, but precious little nutrition.

Eve and I discussed this in earnest during her second visit as she told me she'd tried one weight-loss program after another. "I don't understand how I can still be this overweight and weak," she said, the pain apparent in her voice. "What am I doing wrong?"

I reassured Eve that because people with fibro hurt, they're mostly inactive and thus don't burn calories. And with lack of regular use, muscles quickly become deconditioned and lose strength.

Then I walked her through the eating plan outlined in this chapter, emphasizing that most physicians aren't even aware that food sensitivities—especially gluten sensitivity—can exacerbate fibro symptoms. The same goes for eating "fast carbs" (also called high-glycemic carbs), the kind in white and refined wheat bread, white rice, white pasta, and anything that converts quickly to sugar—hence "fast" in fast carbs.

The sudden blood sugar rise from eating these foods triggers your body to release insulin and plummets your blood sugar, like the first dip of a roller coaster ride. This is called reactive hypoglycemia and is itself a stressor, tightening muscles, exhausting adrenal glands, and worsening further your already stressed fibromyalgia state.

"But what *should* I eat?," Eve asked. "Real food, whole food," I responded. "A bowl of fresh blueberries rather than the pastry-wrapped purple goo they market as blueberry pie. An orange instead of an orange-flavored something. Replacing sugar and junky processed foods with veggies, fruit, 100% whole grains, legumes, and high-quality protein and dairy infuses you with fibro-healing vitamins and minerals, especially B complex, magnesium, and vitamin D."

A definitely thinner and more vibrant Eve began to appear in follow-up visits, clearly pleased with her personal approach to fibro-friendly eating. "I've started cooking like my grandma did," she announced one day, smiling.

I was impressed. How was it going?

"It's going great!" she enthused. "I finally figured out your list of serotonin-boosting foods is like a roadmap, so I loaded up my fridge with fruit and veggies, eggs, fish, and good meats. Started trying the whole grains and legumes and looked up on the internet how to cook them—they're really easy and I portion everything out to freeze and microwave when I need them.

"But you know what really made the difference? Eating protein with every meal and snack. Fruit and yogurt for breakfast—sometimes hard-boiled eggs. Giant salad for lunch, with some cooked meat. A massive plate of cut-up raw vegetables and a few nuts every single day at 4 o'clock, when I used to crave sugar. It keeps me going until dinner, when I pull out some bean or vegetable soup I make on the weekends and freeze. My salads are becoming famous and I even make my own dressings. You know what? I love making my own food and I can't believe how much better I feel."

There's more good news. Eating well gave Eve the energy to start back on a regular walking program, and she's just started lifting light weights. Last time our nurse weighed her she'd lost 15 pounds and looked like a new person, her fibro quickly receding in the rearview mirror.

Part One: Eat to Maximize Internal Serotonin Production

People with fibromyalgia generally are on the low end of measurable serotonin levels, rendering them more susceptible than others to the effects of stress. To invigorate this feel-good neurotransmitter, you'll focus on foods containing tryptophan, which transforms to serotonin in your brain.

The following list shows high-tryptophan foods. Choose richly from it at every meal to generate a steady supply of serotonin, which will keep your mood up and the stress protection of serotonin working for you and your fibro.

As a bonus, eating these high-tryptophan foods will balance the action of your hormones and bolster your resistance to disease by charging up your immune system...because these foods are packed with nutrients your body craves.

Rich sources of tryptophan include protein foods—eat some at every meal:
- All seafood, red meat, chicken, turkey, and soybeans (including tofu), cheese, eggs, yogurt.

More good sources:
- Seeds and nuts, including peanut butter and other nut butters (choose nuts and nut butters with few, if any, added ingredients).
- Dairy foods such as milk, cheese, yogurt, and cottage cheese.
- Lentils and all beans (black, kidney, garbanzo, pinto, etc.)

Look at the buffet of tryptophan-containing produce:

- Broccoli, bananas, cauliflower, asparagus, apricots, cucumbers, kale, tomatoes, Brussels sprouts, green beans, chard, turnip greens, collards, mustard greens, mushrooms, spinach, onions, eggplant, bell peppers, beets, winter squash, garlic, seaweed, and cabbage.

Tryptophan containing grains? Glad you asked:

- Brown rice, oats, barley, and quinoa.

Interestingly, studies show that when healthy people are deliberately placed on tryptophan-free diets, their serotonin levels plummet and they develop symptoms including depression. But the symptoms reverse once they start eating foods containing tryptophan again.

Use this to your advantage by making tryptophan-rich food choices that turn every meal and snack into good-mood food. Tryptophan also helps limit carb cravings and will regulate your appetite.

A little background on how tryptophan turns to serotonin

Tryptophan is one of a group of molecules known as amino acids, the building blocks of proteins. Once in your brain, tryptophan changes to 5 hydroxytryptophan (5HTP for short) and then to serotonin. Along the way, these reactions require B vitamins (found in virtually all tryptophan foods), especially vitamin B-6 and certain healthy fats—specifically the omega-3s in fish, walnuts, and grass-fed beef.

With these nutritional components in place, your brain becomes an efficient serotonin-manufacturing enterprise with one final assist. In order to transport tryptophan to your brain, you need insulin. And to get insulin, you need to eat carbohydrates. (But please keep reading because some carbs are decidedly better than others.)

When you eat carbs, they're broken down into various sugars and as they're absorbed into your bloodstream they alert the pancreas to release insulin, which carries tryptophan into your brain. And there it's converted to serotonin.

"Fast" carbs vs high-quality carbohydrates
You've seen how carbohydrates work to increase your shaky levels of serotonin. But various carbs are handled differently by your body. On one side we have the highly refined, "fast" carbs (fast because they're quickly digested and turned to sugar) of foods such as white rice, white-flour pasta and bakery goods, white and refined wheat bread, crackers, chips, cookies, cakes, candy, fruit juice, and soda — all highly processed foods and, for those familiar with the Glycemic Index, all high-GI foods.

True, these fast carbs will help tryptophan get to your brain, but they also dramatically raise and then plummet your blood sugar, which your body perceives as stress. You don't need more stress, period. Put simply: stress boosts adrenal hormone output, leading to increased cortisol release and accumulation of belly fat. Stand up and look down in the general direction of your toes. If your belly's in the way, you're likely eating too many fast carbs.

And here's why carb cravings come in cycles. Eating fast carbs (as opposed to, say, half a cup of kidney bean salad with veggies and a few cheese cubes) boosts your blood sugar so quickly you feel a "high" before the crash. Then, insulin kicks in, plummeting your blood sugar, you're hungry enough to eat your desk...and the cycle starts all over again.

Instead, focus on high-quality complex carbs, the ones found in fruit, nuts, vegetables, beans, and 100% whole grains (more on these below). High-quality carbohydrates deliver lots of fiber, vitamins, minerals, and other nutrients per serving, along with a rock-steady supply of insulin. Enjoy some complex carbs at every meal and snack throughout your day.

The fundamental difference between the two types of carbs is their chemical structure, but we're most interested in the fact that complex carbs are loaded with fiber, which means they take longer to digest, sending your blood sugar and serotonin on a nice slow ride upward—with no blood sugar crash—and keeping you feeling fuller longer.

Ten Easy Ways to Boost Serotonin

1. **Eat dark leafy greens four times a week.** Purchase spinach, kale, swiss chard, and collards (available fresh or pre-washed in bags), chopping and steaming them for a few minutes before tossing them with flavorful additions such as a glug of olive oil, a spritz of lemon, chopped herbs, and feta cheese. Olives, too, and some cooked meat (high in tryptophan) or hard-boiled eggs. Chop raw kale into coleslaw, steam chard ribbons and use as a bed for chicken.

2. **Have a little protein with every meal and snack.** Choose from a variety of tryptophan-rich proteins—from eggs, fish, chicken, pork, and beef to cheese, peanut and other nut butters, and quinoa. You need protein regularly, but you don't need a lot of it. Enjoy a palm-

sized portion of any red meat, fish, or chicken every day, or combine brown rice and beans to create complete protein. Eggs are an excellent protein source that stand ready to serve at any meal (hard-boiled eggs add protein power to salads, snacks, and sandwiches). Or snack on a slice of high-quality cheese and an apple. Other go-to proteins include yogurt, cottage cheese, nuts, beans, and lentils. Please make protein choices carefully, though. Farmed fish doesn't have the beneficial omega-3 fats of wild-caught fish because they're fed a grain-based feed, rather than eating plankton. Same goes for factory-farmed meats, which also contain hormones. Choose instead grass-fed beef plus eggs and chickens from a trusted local source. The Environmental Working Group has a handy meat-eater's guide with more on all this (Google "EWG tips for meat eaters").

3. **Never miss a meal or snack.** Skipping meals or light snacks causes dramatic swings in blood sugar and triggers symptoms such as lightheadedness, brain fog, irritability, and tremulousness, all of which are perceived as stress by your fibro-coping body. Low blood sugar can also send you running for whatever food happens to be closest, like nutritionally empty vending machine snacks or the donut box sitting out at work. Keep high-quality carbs on hand at home and at work — vegetable soups, nuts, fruit, raw veggies, and 100% whole-grain bread (such as Ezekiel bread) with a little cheese or natural peanut butter — to prevent toppling into a blood sugar valley. Most important, base breakfast, lunch, and dinner on the suggestions in this chapter, with protein and complex carbohydrates (fruits, veggies, nuts, and whole grains), and you'll avoid the valleys altogether.

4. **Have a salad five days a week.** Look for the darkest salad greens you can find — they contain the most nutrients. Good choices include dark green romaine and red leaf lettuces, and also one of my favorite fast foods, pre-washed organic baby spinach. Once your greens are in the bowl, get creative: add walnuts, a little intensely favored cheese (such as feta or bleu), and whatever else appeals — blueberries, sliced pear, or strawberries are lovely for one effect, red onion, sweet pepper, and tomato for another. Whisk together an olive oil and vinegar dressing and toss. You can get an enormous about of veggies into a single bowl, and don't forget the high-tryptophan add-ins: cooked hot or cold chicken or other meats, canned tuna or salmon, or a handful of drained kidney or garbanzo beans. Or sauté some ground turkey with onion, oregano, and basil and add it hot to your greens before tossing in the veggies. Cooked veggies add diversity. Dice a couple of baby eggplant, sauté in olive oil until soft, and toss them in. Chopped hard-boiled eggs are a mainstay protein addition to salads.

5. **One night a week, make it veggie night.** Raw or cooked, veggie night can include washed and cut raw radishes, carrots, sweet peppers of every color, and a cruciferous vegetable like broccoli or cauliflower. Try baby zucchini or yellow squash raw, sliced lengthwise. Experiment with dips. Make an easy bean dip by putting a can of white beans, red beans, or black beans into the blender with some garlic, fresh lemon juice, a little tahini, and a few drops of olive oil. Shake in any spices that appeal, such as oregano or basil. Salsas make delicious dips too. Make a creamy salsa dip by adding a tablespoon or two of sour cream to red or green salsa. Or enjoy your

vegetables hot, by steaming them, draining, and tossing with olive oil and some grated intensely flavored cheese (parmesan, bleu, sharp cheddar) and fresh herbs. A couple tablespoons of peanut butter whisked with an equal amount of lime juice and soy sauce make a satisfying sauce over steamed broccoli or cauliflower. For dessert, enjoy fruit or a small piece of dark chocolate.

6. **Make eggs** Eggs are an exceptional source of protein (needed to generate tryptophan, from which serotonin is made), easy to prepare, and versatile enough to have for breakfast, lunch, or dinner.

7. **Enjoy nuts** Great for snacks and adding to salads, nuts are a high-quality carbohydrate that contain protein, disease-fighting antioxidants, and health-giving oils. They're an ideal food and especially delicious when combined with fruit or tossed into green salads. Enjoy one third cup of any nut every day.

8. **Become a soup lover** Make a big batch of bean or vegetable soup and enjoy as a snack or for lunch or dinner. Soup is enormously satisfying and will give you a carbohydrate/serotonin lift.

9. **Lean on legumes** Here's a powerful feel-good food with an antioxidant, mineral, and fiber content that makes them exceptional for everyday eating. Start looking at your grocery shelf in a new way and experiment with all types of canned legumes — kidney beans, garbanzo beans (chickpeas), butter beans, lentils. Drain, warm them, and add olive oil and spices. Add meat or not. Enjoy cold as a salad by tossing with an olive oil and vinegar dressing, chopped sweet peppers, and some cubed Swiss cheese. You can buy all types of legumes already hydrated in cans — this is one prepared food I heartily endorse. Or

you can rehydrate them yourself by cooking from their dried state. Incredibly versatile, legumes are an ideal choice for serotonin boosting.

10. **Stop dieting and start eating real food.** Quit the junky, processed diet foods! The best way to pump up serotonin, improve your health, and lose weight is to eat the widest possible range of high-quality plant foods along with protein. If you're struggling with what that means, return to the top of this section and review the list again.

Got the concept? Good. Now you're going to apply "raising your serotonin" eating to…

Part Two: Eat foods free of toxins and other environmental contaminants

Your low serotonin renders you more sensitive than others to chemicals in the environment. This means you not only have a greater sensitivity to medications and scents like perfumes and glues, but also to the numerous chemicals added to manufactured food and to the pesticides on non-organic fruits and veggies.

Getting rid of these toxins as completely as possible will be easy for some people and more difficult for others, especially anyone addicted to chemical-laced foods like diet colas and most prepared foods. Over the past 20 years, it's alarming the number of women who have told me "I'm really addicted to diet cola" and literally go through an uncomfortable withdrawal period when they stop it.

Eliminate processed and fast foods

The easiest way to eliminate toxins is to stop eating the

chemical swill of processed, prepared, and fast foods. How to accomplish this? Start making your own food from fruits, vegetables, high-quality meats and eggs, and organic 100% whole grains.

Begin today reducing and then eliminating all fast foods, including prepared meals (unless you know and feel comfortable with the source). Leading this category are most of the so-called meals you find in the grocery freezer — the cuisines in a box that are "lean" only because they contain miniscule portions of actual food. Take a magnifying glass next time you shop and you'll see the ingredients for most of these tiny (and expensive) dinners make up one long list of chemical additives. Read the ingredient list aloud. If you can't pronounce an ingredient, return the box to the shelf or freezer, remembering how easy it is to say, "Whole grains, tomatoes, and even bok choy."

These highly processed "meals" are brought to you by agribusiness conglomerates that create this junk and market it heavily to time-pressed, weight-conscious, and nutrient-starved women. If your body could talk it might say, "What are you trying to do to me with this stuff?" Instead, it speaks the language of fibro: low energy, weight gain, unhealthy-looking skin and hair.

When you start eating food with actual nutrients you'll feel better and look better.

Trust me, your body knows the difference between real food and junky food and drink, which contain a lot of nasty, health-destroying refined flours, sugar (including high-fructose corn syrup), salt, and fats like hydrogenated oils. And significantly, processing itself removes most nutrients from food.

How do I get started eating real food?

Read Part 1 on maximizing internal serotonin production for ideas. Here are a few more:

Steam a large portion of any vegetable—spinach, cauliflower, broccoli, kale, summer squash, green beans—and add a couple tablespoons of olive oil, some herbs (dry or fresh), a little acid (vinegar, lemon, or lime), and a crumbling of intensely flavored cheese (feta, bleu, pecorino). Toss in a cooked and sliced chicken breast or thigh. By cooking meats on the weekend, slicing, and freezing, you'll eat easily all week long. Add a few kidney beans and you've got a near-perfect meal.

Your body—and fibro—will thank you. That's because instead of chemicals, *you are eating real food.*

For lunch, toss the darkest greens you can find—spinach, baby kale, romaine—with a hard-boiled egg and a some tuna for protein, plus raw or cooked veggies and a few walnuts. Whisk together a dressing of Dijon mustard, olive oil, and vinegar. Take this to work. Don't get a carry-out salad—you wouldn't believe the manufactured food they use at most carry-out places.

To further avoid toxins, choose meat that doesn't come from factory farms. All those hormones and antibiotics. Am I aiming for your wallet? Not at all. Just eat smaller portions of responsibly raised quality meat (grass-fed beef, hormone-free chickens—available at Whole Foods) or choose alternative protein sources. Many groceries now carry eggs laid by chickens that have lived a free-range, additive-free life. Google "EWG tips for meat eaters" to read the Environmental Working Group's meat-eater's guide.

Some organic frozen meals contain mostly actual food.

Become a label reader and you'll see what I mean. It's still less expensive to make your own, though. Get some Ezekiel tortillas (made with 100% whole grain), warm up some black beans, mash an avocado, chop cilantro and a tomato, and get out the salsa.

Virtually every boxed grain product contains chemicals you don't need. Start shopping the dry bins at Whole Foods or your health food store, helping yourself to healthful whole grains including brown rice, oatmeal, and quinoa (dried beans and legumes too). Cook large batches on the weekend and freeze in half-cup portions to pull out during the week ahead.

It's OK to purchase canned beans, canned fish like tuna and salmon, and canned tomatoes. These are your new convenience foods.

If you're curious to see how sensitive your body is to chemicals, try this experiment. After you've been squeaky-clean and chemical-free for a couple of months, eat a full meal of chemical-laden food—a bag of Cheetos, a Big Mac, a diet Coke, store-bought cole slaw, or a dinner in a box. See how your body responds. Be assured you won't want to repeat this experiment twice.

What you'll feel if you try this is a common detoxification phenomenon that demonstrates how efficiently your body can numb itself after repeated exposure to a toxin. The most dramatic example occurs with cigarettes. The very first time you smoke, your body screams "Don't do this!" by making you feel really ill. But after a few weeks, the cigarettes not only disconnect this warning system, but convert it into an addiction. When you quit anything (cigarettes, diet colas, white-flour carbs, sugar) you're resetting your warning system to start working again.

Just like if you've ever smoked, stopped for a year, and then succumbed to temptation and lit up "just one" you probably felt like you were going to throw up. That's the reset of your warning system. The same phenomenon will occur if you reintroduce toxic, chemically laced food into your pristine body.

Purchasing chemical-free produce

Along with reading labels (and not eating much food with a label at all) and avoiding foods with artificial colors, additives, preservatives, and hormones, your best strategy for eating free of toxins and chemicals is to buy organic produce.

The Environmental Working Group again can help you be even smarter about your choices. Their Shopper's Guide to Pesticides in Produce is available online. Here are the highlights:

Dirty Dozen, containing the most pesticide residue. Purchase these organic.

1. Apples
2. Celery
3. Strawberries
4. Peaches
5. Spinach
6. Nectarines, imported
7. Grapes, imported
8. Sweet bell peppers
9. Potatoes
10. Blueberries, domestic
11. Lettuce
12. Kale/collard greens

Clean 15, lowest in pesticides. These are OK to purchase non-organic.

1. Onions
2. Sweet corn
3. Pineapple
4. Avocado
5. Asparagus
6. Sweet peas
7. Mangoes
8. Eggplant
9. Cantaloupe, domestically grown
10. Kiwi
11. Cabbage
12. Watermelon
13. Sweet potatoes
14. Grapefruit
15. Mushrooms

Purchasing organic produce was once an enormously expensive undertaking and it depressed me that healthful eating was available only for people who had a lot of money to spend. However, I was cheered when I saw that Walmart was adding substantial amounts of fresh organic foods to their shelves. A taste comparison published in Atlantic Monthly Magazine even found (to their surprise) that the quality of the Walmart produce was largely equal to that at Whole Foods, where you can easily go broke in the produce section.

A word about cost

I hear it all the time from my patients: fresh produce costs a lot, not to mention organic! Let's do some comparison shopping. At my local chain grocery, potato chips (a food devoid of nutrients) cost between $4 and $4.50 per pound. One type of crunchy cinnamon breakfast cereal (another virtually empty food whose ingredient list includes highly refined rice flour and three types of sugar: white sugar, fructose, and dextrose) costs $5.00 per pound. Even a so-called 100% natural cereal made by one of the food giants contains partially hydrogenated cottonseed oil (nothing natural or good for you about trans-fats) and comes in at just under $5.00 per pound.

Contrast this to washed baby spinach at $4.96 per pound, but with nutrients galore. Popcorn, at 50 to 75 cents per pound, is the original snack food you make yourself. Natural peanut and other nut butters are excellent protein sources and also a fine carb snack on 100% whole grain Ezekiel bread, tucked into celery, or smeared on apple slices. They run about $4 per pound.

At the low end of the expense scale (and the high end of the nutrient scale) is all manner of fresh produce. A 2004 US Department of Agriculture (USDA) study found that three servings of fresh fruit and four servings of fresh vegetables cost about 64 cents. To my knowledge the study hasn't been updated, but even if this number increased it would still be a grand bargain.

It's true that some out-of-season fruits and veggies run more, and that's why shopping in season is the way to go. In the summer, visit the farmers market for fresh corn, tomatoes, peppers, and squash and make a meal of them.

Even if we doubled the USDA figure to accommodate your higher servings of vegetables and fruits, your total daily expense is about $1.25…still far less than a chemical-laden Frappuccino.

And now that you've learned to raise your serotonin and detoxify yourself, let's move on to a very important aspect of fibro-friendly eating...

Part Three: Uncover and Eliminate Potential Food Sensitivities

It's quite possible you're sensitive to certain foods themselves, chemically free or not. Let me emphasize that this isn't the same as being allergic to a food, like the people whose lips swell when they eat strawberries or throats close up after nibbling seafood or peanuts.

Food sensitivities are more subtle, producing vague symptoms such as fatigue, muscle pain, and bloating.

Also, because these symptoms can occur a day or two *after* you eat the offending food, food sensitivities are usually more challenging to uncover. Doctors aren't exactly sure how food sensitivities produce symptoms, but the current thinking centers on a controversial diagnosis called leaky gut syndrome, in which culprit foods "leak" through your intestinal wall, triggering your immune system to create antibodies against them. The combination of food molecules and antibodies then triggers low levels of inflammation, which in turn produces a stress response and a variety of seemingly unrelated symptoms.

You don't need undiscovered food sensitivities adding more stress to your fibro. In this section you'll become a detective. It's a two-step process:

1. Start the Food Sensitivity Elimination-Reintroduction Eating Program. I walk you through it just below on page 167. It takes about a month and is very much worth the effort. If your health insurance covers blood tests for food sensitivities that's a bonus, but remember: how you feel when you eliminate and then reintroduce potential culprit foods always takes precedence over any blood test results.

2. If it turns out that wheat is one of your culprit foods, ask your doctor to order a blood test for gluten sensitivity. Gluten is a type of protein found in many grains (wheat, barley, rye, some oats, kamut, and triticale) and, by extension, in many cereals and breads and a slew of processed foods. If you're sensitive to gluten, your immune system has created an antibody against the gluten molecule, and these antibodies circulate in your bloodstream, triggering widespread (and stressful) inflammation.

A blood test will show if your immune system is creating antibodies against gluten. As a rule of thumb, anytime your body creates antibodies against anything, the message is that your body is trying to get rid of it. If you have a positive test result for gluten, your doctor may refer you to a gastroenterologist, who will take a biopsy of your small intestine (this sounds much worse than it actually is) that can show damage being caused by the gluten molecule.

Gluten sensitivity won a "dubious achievement" award from internists some years back as being the most overlooked diagnosis causing chronic symptoms. Physicians began to appreciate there were many more problems linked to gluten sensitivity than the full-blown characteristic intestinal malabsorption of celiac disease. These gluten sensitivity problems include skin rashes, joint pain, neurologic and psychiatric conditions, and symptoms like fatigue, anxiety, and headaches. In fact, an article in the *New England Journal of Medicine* listed 55 conditions that could be caused by a gluten-sensitive person regularly eating gluten.

When patients discover they're gluten-sensitive and eliminate it from their lives, their overall sense of well-being skyrockets. This is especially true for fibro patients.

If your blood test is negative but you know you felt a lot better off gluten, please listen to the wisdom of your body and don't guide your decision-making based on the test. The longstanding symptoms you'd been experiencing were messages of distress. By quitting gluten, you responded to the message and your body rewarded you with a new sense of well-being. After hearing a message as loud as that, ignoring it by going back on gluten is like taking the phone off the hook when someone is calling to let you know your house is on fire.

Ask Dr E: Why is it so important to determine if I'm gluten sensitive?

- If you have chronic symptoms of virtually any kind (digestive, musculoskeletal, dermatological, psychiatric, neurological—anything chronic), if gluten sensitivity is contributing to them you'll never feel completely well until you eliminate gluten.

- Since we eat an astonishing amount of gluten grains (many people eat gluten-containing foods at every meal and for snacks), the total number of gluten-sensitive people, estimated to be in the millions, is rising dramatically and—here's the kicker—99% of them are undiagnosed.

- If you don't figure out a possible gluten connection, you'll be in and out of the doctor's office frequently with vague symptoms, your doctor saying she can't find anything wrong with you, that your tests are normal. This is because gluten sensitivity testing is simply not routinely done (though it should be).

- If you're gluten sensitive and you keep eating gluten, you won't live as long.

Food Sensitivity Elimination-Reintroduction Eating Program

This self-test will help you discover whether certain foods are making your fibro worse. Remember, you're in charge of interpreting your body's response — no doctors telling you how you feel. This is all about you and your food.

Most of my patients set up a calendar that lays out the bones of this program. That way you won't find yourself at dinner wondering if it's OK to have cheese. In fact, getting ready for this takes a little advance planning and sticking to it requires a bit of discipline, but I know you're up to it and the results will be worth the effort.

The most common food irritants are dairy and wheat. If dairy is setting you off, you may have lactose intolerance, a problem digesting the milk sugar lactose. However, this is not the same as dairy sensitivity via the leaky gut model I explained earlier. You can have them both: lactose intolerance *and* dairy sensitivity.

Days 1-14

Eliminate all foods in the six food groups most commonly linked to food sensitivities. If you're still eating prepared foods, you'll have to read labels to check for ingredients that include any of the six, which are:

- **Dairy products**, including milk, cream, yogurt (dairy-

167

free probiotics are available at health food stores), ice cream, sour cream, and cheese. If it comes from a cow or a goat, eliminate it.

- **Eggs**, including all foods containing eggs.
- **Corn** and corn products.
- **Citrus** Easy to spot: orange, lemon, lime, grapefruit, tangerine, etc.
- **Soy** and all products containing it. I added soy to this program just last year after seeing more and more people reacting adversely to it.
- **Wheat** and all the gluten grains (barley, rye, oats, kamut, triticale). Definitely the most difficult to eliminate, since wheat is found not just in obvious places (bread, baked goods, and all flours not labeled gluten-free), but also in packaged soups, dressings, soy sauce, fake crab meat, some veggie burgers, sauces, beer, and more.

Now before you imploringly ask, "But what am I going to eat?" believe me, no one has ever starved to death with full access to all grains except the gluten group. Remember brown rice? Barley? Buckwheat? Quinoa? This is a good opportunity to try some new whole grains. Also, you can eat all vegetables, potatoes, meat, poultry, fish, and fruit (except citrus), which will start you on the path to eating the whole foods this plan is centered on. You might grieve being deprived of your fettuccine Alfredo (the trifecta of culprit foods—dairy, egg and wheat), but you'll not die without it.

As you move through the program, you might be surprised to discover how much you eat from one particular group. For example, many people eat products containing wheat (waffles, pancakes, doughnuts, scones, bread, muffins, pasta—even whole-grain versions) several times a day for years on end.

After you've eliminated the six food groups for two weeks, do a body scan.

Do you sense an improvement in any of your longstanding symptoms or a general sense of feeling better? If you feel exactly the same after two weeks of food elimination as you did before, you probably don't have an issue with food sensitivities and you can begin to eat an unrestricted diet of the delicious foods laid out in this chapter.

If, however, one or more of your symptoms has improved or you just generally feel better, you may be onto something important. "Better" is, of course, vague, but it's your body and you're the one most intimately acquainted with how you feel. For you, "better" may mean less gas and bloating, less muscle aching and fatigue, clearer sinuses, anything.

Now start the reintroduction phase one food group at a time, as follows:

Days 15-18: Re-introduce dairy in any quantity you're comfortable with. Monitor yourself for a return of any symptoms. If none appear, dairy isn't a problem and you can return to eating dairy and move on to reintroducing the next food group. If, however, some symptoms return, stop having dairy altogether.

Days 19-21: Reintroduce eggs, watching carefully for symptoms. If you do have symptoms, stop eating eggs. If you have no symptoms, continue to eat eggs and move on to the next group, paying attention every step of the way to how you feel.

Days 22-24: Reintroduce corn.

Days 25-27: Reintroduce soy.

Days 28-30: Reintroduce citrus.

Days 31-33: Reintroduce wheat and the other gluten grains.

Over these weeks of restriction and reintroduction I hope you'll learn something about how your body responds to the foods you eat. A new patient I'll call Holly told me this story: She'd had a nasty peeling rash the size of a walnut on her foot and after a year of trying various remedies, including the ones prescribed by a dermatologist, in an unrelated-to-the-foot effort to lose weight she eliminated most flour-based foods (bread, cake, cookies, crackers) from her diet.

Not only did Holly lose 25 pounds over the next few months, but her foot rash cleared completely. A gluten sensitivity? Probably. She can tolerate gluten in small amounts now, though she saves it for very special occasions.

Like Holly, understand you'll not necessarily be off any culprit food for the rest of your life. If you discover, for example, that dairy causes symptoms, start a fresh 12-week break from it and then gradually reintroduce it, along with any other culprit foods, on a rotational basis.

Plan to eat one of the culprit foods twice weekly, say Monday and Thursday, but never at the same time as another culprit food. Meaning: if dairy and wheat are symptom triggers, take a 12-week break from both, and then allow yourself dairy Mondays and Thursdays, wheat on Tuesdays and Fridays. The only exception to this is if you have a definite diagnosis of celiac disease (by blood test and biopsy). In that case, you'll need to give up gluten altogether.

Ask Dr E: What Symptoms Can be Caused
By Food Sensitivities?

I'm glad you asked, because with food sensitivity symptoms it's not just your digestive system talking back. All kinds of symptoms are linked to food sensitivities. Take a look at the list, keeping in mind that most of these have more than one cause, with food sensitivity a relatively common and frequently overlooked one.

To investigate your symptoms further, try the Food Sensitivity Elimination-Reintroduction Eating Program.

- **General** Fatigue, anxiety, depression, insomnia, food cravings, weight gain.

- **Infections** Recurring colds, urinary tract infections, sore throats, ear infections, yeast infections.

- **Ear, Nose, and Throat** Chronic nasal congestion, postnasal drip, fluid in the ears, Ménière's syndrome (which can include vertigo, hearing loss, ear pressure, and ringing in the ear).

- **Gastrointestinal** Irritable bowel syndrome, constipation, diarrhea, abdominal cramping, ulcerative colitis, Crohn's disease, gallbladder disease.

- **Cardiovascular** High blood pressure, irregular heartbeat, angina.

- **Dermatologic** Acne, eczema, psoriasis, canker sores, hives.

- **Rheumatologic** Muscle aches, osteoarthritis, rheumatoid arthritis.

- **Neurologic** Migraines and other headaches, focus and concentration problems, numbness and tingling of the hands and feet.

- **Miscellaneous** Asthma, frequent urination, teeth grinding, bedwetting, infantile colic.

Part 4: Eat to Avoid Hypoglycemia (Low Blood Sugar) and Adrenal Fatigue

Hypoglycemia isn't a food sensitivity or allergy, but it stresses your already fibro-stressed system and it's definitely linked to focus and concentration problems. Your brain simply can't tolerate low blood sugar. Ever know someone who literally became irrational when she skipped a meal?

Low blood sugar is the most common cause of adrenal stress. Considering that adrenal fatigue is one of the most significant sources of the fatigue that accompanies your fibromyalgia, you want to be good to your adrenals and not worry them by placing yourself at risk of hypoglycemia. Any time your blood sugar is unusually low, your whole body regards the situation as a MAJOR EMERGENCY. The same cascade of events occur as if you'd been attacked by a mugger. The outpouring adrenalin mobilizes sugar stores in your muscles and liver, but in the process of this heroic rescue your muscles tighten up.

Do you, as a person with fibro, actually need your muscles tightened even further?

Our bodies undergo this 911 alarm any time our blood sugar is low because we're genetically hard-wired to provide a constant state of nutrition to our brains.

My late father-in-law, a generally mild and likable fellow, turned into an ogre whenever he skipped a meal. He wasn't diabetic, but everyone in our family could recognize the first signs of his hypoglycemia. This led to immediate scrabbling around in various purses for something — anything — to feed him, not unlike the carnivorous plant Audrey in "Little Shop of Horrors," who also didn't like being hypoglycemic. Diabetics who've experienced hypoglycemia report rapid heart rate, mental confusion, sweating, and shakiness — in fact, all the symptoms of an adrenalin surge (and a panic attack). The result of these hypoglycemic episodes? Muscle tightness and adrenal fatigue.

By merely increasing protein and reducing high-glycemic foods, you can easily treat hypoglycemia yourself. To keep your blood sugar stable, vastly reduce (or eliminate altogether if you're gluten-sensitive) foods made from white flour, which is what's left after wheat flour is refined to remove the bran and fiber, the nutritional good guys. White-flour products enter your bloodstream almost as quickly as sugar, spiking your blood sugar instead of taking it on a slow ride upward. When your blood sugar crashes a short time later, you're shaky and hungry again. Eating high-quality carbohydrates (see page 152) generates an evenly paced blood sugar rise. These good carbs also help your body make serotonin.

Threats to blood sugar stability

Blood sugar crashers include white flour foods and other refined foods such as white rice and non-100% whole grain breads, pastries, cookies, baked good, and pasta. Reserve for very special occasions your intake of bakery goods (donuts, cakes, pies, and cookies) and crackers, all of which are also common vehicles for trans-fats and saturated fat. Cereals fall into a middle category: some, like steel-cut oats, are very high in fiber and are extremely good for you. Most boxed cereals contain highly refined flours and lots of sugar. Make your own cereal from oats, millet, or barley.

Finding 100% whole-grain products, which don't aggravate blood sugar, can be challenging. Choose brown or wild rice over white. For bread, make your mainstay a 100% whole-grain version like Ezekiel bread, available in the freezer section at Whole Foods and other groceries. Don't be fooled by marketing labels boasting a bread is "multigrain," "whole wheat," or "made with whole grains." They are not 100% whole grain.

Always check the ingredients: if you see "whole wheat flour" on the list, consider the bread made with whole wheat grains. But if you see "flour" or "wheat flour," know that this is refined flour, stripped of its nutrition. Cooking your own whole grains is the most reliable way to go. Try wheat berries, millet, and teff, all easily prepared in large batches. Freeze into half-cup portions and enjoy them throughout the week with protein.

To seriously stabilize your blood sugar, you need to eat actual food for each meal and for snacks (see Part 1 of this chapter for guidance). No dipping into the crackers, chips, or ice cream. Health-giving, blood sugar-stabilizing snacks include carrots and a hard-boiled egg, an apple and a piece of cheese, or a pear and a few walnuts. Remember, eating protein keeps your blood sugar stable.

Serious threats to blood sugar should be obvious: skipping meals is the worst offender. People can inadvertently bring this on themselves when they attempt a cleansing fast or a juice-only detoxification (juice is mainly sugar, remember?).

And while low blood sugar is the most serious threat to our adrenals, caffeine is a close second. A modest amount of caffeine, especially in the morning, is harmless. By evening, the caffeine will have pretty well metabolized out of your body and won't interfere with sleep. But treating afternoon fatigue with caffeine ("I need an extra-shot Starbucks to make it to dinner") is asking for adrenal tsuris. Envision a slave ship. The poor slaves rowing under the whip of the slavedriver are your adrenals. The guy with the whip? That's afternoon caffeine.

Ask Dr E: Is Breakfast Really So Important? I'm Not Hungry in the Morning.

Breakfast is so essential I could write a whole book on it but won't. I'll just nag you like your mother once did. Breakfast literally reminds us that we're "breaking the fast," eating for the first time since we went to sleep.

For people with fibro, it's especially vital to eat a daily breakfast and eat one that will sustain your blood sugar at least until a midmorning snack. Otherwise you're just laying more stress on top of fibro stress as your body cries out for nutrients on which it can run.

Since you're not hungry when you wake up, try to eat part of your breakfast within an hour of waking, saving the rest for a couple of hours later when your appetite improves.

Breaking away from traditional breakfast foods might also pique your interest. If time's short in the morning, prepare something the night before. Try half a natural peanut butter sandwich on 100% whole-grain bread (such as the Ezekiel brand) with an apple on the side. Add sliced banana or chopped prunes to your sandwich. Or load your whole-grain bread with cold sliced turkey or chicken, half an avocado, and fresh baby spinach.

Since you're practicing portion control to keep your weight in check, you could easily have leftovers from last night's dinner for breakfast. The world will not come crashing down if you warm up half a pork chop to accompany a pair of hard boiled eggs. A combination like this will keep your blood sugar as level and steady as the mind of a meditating Buddhist monk.

Protein's essential and eggs are a fine source. Keep hard-boiled eggs in the fridge to eat with a piece of cheese and a pear. Or cook an omelet, adding mushrooms, onion, spinach, (or any veggies) and a little cheese. You can easily make omelets the night before and microwave it in the morning.

The champion of breakfast cereals—oatmeal—is another top choice (as is its sister whole grain, barley). Add protein-laden milk, nuts, or yogurt on top, along with fruit and ground flaxseed. A cup of oatmeal contains soluble fiber and also phytochemicals called flavonoids—antioxidants that are key to disease prevention. Because your body digests oatmeal slowly, your serotonin moves upward slowly, keeping blood sugar even. Cook a batch of steel-cut oats on the weekend and portion out a week's daily half-cup supply into small bowls in the fridge. Then, just microwave, add the extras, and enjoy. If you can't get to it before leaving, eat a piece of fruit and cheese and take your oatmeal to work.

Here's another night-before idea: cut up a variety of fruits on top of a cup of plain yogurt or cottage cheese. Stash in the fridge and the next day sprinkle with cinnamon and enjoy.

By the way, when researchers took a survey of people who had made it to age 100, the single most consistent trait among them was that they never missed breakfast. Plus, while breakfast keeps your blood sugar stable on the way to a healthy old age, you'll simply feel better all day long for having eaten it.

Now, armed with all this information on eating to raise your serotonin and reduce stress, here's what everyone really cares about…

Part Five: Eat to Prevent Weight Gain…and Encourage Weight Loss

You're probably overweight. Nothing personal. I can't see you but it's a fact that the vast majority of people with fibro accumulate pounds. Don't feel "why me?" about this. Any normal-weight person who became too tired to function, had 24/7 painful muscles, and craved sugary carbs because they made her vaguely "feel better" would inevitably gain weight.

If you've eagerly jumped to this section before reading the rest of the chapter, please go back and read it now, including Eve's story right at the beginning. You'll quickly see that just by eliminating junky foods and foods you're sensitive to, that contain chemicals, that are processed, and that spike blood sugar you'll be rewarded for your efforts with a nice steady weight loss. The foods that boost feel-good serotonin (Part 1) are a mini-meal plan themselves for weight loss. Go ahead and read it now—I'll be here when you get back.

As you clean up your eating, your pain will relent and your energy will surge. At that point you can start can burning calories by being more physically active and your weight will drop further. In his book *The False Fat Diet*, Elson M. Haas, MD, describes how eating foods you're sensitive to promotes intercellular fluid retention and weight gain (hence the "false fat"), so this aspect alone should trigger a prompt weight reduction.

But there's a caveat here because another real villain of weight gain or lack of weight loss is forgetting to cut portion size. What's most vital is reducing your calorie intake, but remember there's still a lot of healthful foods you can and should be eating. Raw veggies and fruit are free, and by being careful with portions of the other whole foods in this plan—meats, nuts, legumes, whole grains—you'll see results, I promise.

Mastering the art of portion control

These seven steps will help you on your way. Gentle reminder: gratefully enjoy every mouthful you eat.

1. **Donate all 11-inch plates to a resale shop.** Never eat another meal off anything larger than a 9-inch plate and you'll immediately reduce calories by 20%.

2. **When you're done preparing a meal, place portions on your 9-inch plates** and leftovers in the fridge (nothing like cold food to chill a desire for seconds).

3. **Never bring a serving platter to the table** unless it's piled high with fresh fruit and veggies. These are "free" foods you can—and should—load up on daily.

4. **Read all labels** and never buy or eat any food containing refined wheat flour, white flour, or high fructose corn syrup. In fact, don't buy many foods with labels at all. Your food shouldn't have to explain itself, to justify its existence, before you eat it.

5. **Prepare most of your own food** to avoid the excesses of packaged foods and eating out. Focus on whole foods— fruits, vegetables, legumes, protein, and whole grains.

6. **If you do eat out.** First, return the bread basket to your waiter. Tell him its nothing personal, you just don't need a large basket of refined white flour products and a tub of butter. In Chicago, most servers are quite slim themselves and they'll admire your fortitude. Then, when your meal arrives, immediately divide it in half and ask for half to be wrapped to take home.

7. **Slow down when eating and don't watch TV or read during your meal.** If you eat too quickly, your brain won't get the message that your stomach is full until after you've overeaten. Doing other things while you eat encourages overeating.

Depending on the severity of your weight problem, you may

want to restrict daily calories to 1,200. In general, follow the steps in this chapter, cutting out altogether the cookies, cakes, crackers, fast-carb breads, and other refined foods that are high in calories, low in fiber, and that pack on the pounds. Also, the "diet" foods that are not real food at all.

In addition:

- **Quit the calorie-laden liquids** including all fruit juice (eat whole fruit instead), sodas (diet sodas too), and anything sweetened — tea, coffee, "sports drinks," everything.

- **Exercise regularly** See Week 1 of the Nearly Natural Cure (page 106) for how to begin. Later in that chapter, you'll increase the amount.

- **Stay active** Activities that you may not think of as exercise can be great calorie burners: opt for stairs over elevator, tend your garden, walk, stretch, never sit for longer than 20 minutes, do your computer work standing up. Remember, your goal is to exercise every day you eat.

- **Forget fad diets** They may produce short-term weight loss, but they rarely keep weight off permanently. Aim to lose just one or two pounds a week. When weight comes off at a slow but steady rate, it tends to stay off.

Sugar

It's simply amazing the amount of sugar we're eating these days. By analyzing grocery store lists in pioneer days, apparently we ate about 15 pounds of sugar per year. Now, because sugar is being added to everything from boxed cereal to potato salad (and especially in the form of high fructose corn syrup), we're eating about 150 pounds per year. That's 30 five-pound bags of sugar every year, close to a half a pound of sugar every day.

In addition to quitting soft drinks, fruit juices, and all other sugared drinks, don't add sugar to your food and dramatically cut the sugar-containing foods you eat every day, though by this I certainly don't mean limit fruit. It's a champion at satisfying a sweet tooth, as are sweet potatoes, beets, and carrots, all with nature's own sugars.

Other sugar-containing foods? One of the quickest ways to start losing weight is to cut them out entirely. Oh, by the way, once you do quit sugar, you'll lose your taste for the stuff. Avoid sugar for a month and then tackle a chocolate Dunkin' Donut and dollars to donuts (sorry) you'll say "Yeccch! Too sweet!"

Fibro Quicksand: Keeping "magnetic" foods in your house

We've all been there: a chocolate cake appears for a birthday party or Aunt Fran delivers a tin of her famous cookies. And there are leftovers.

In subsequent days, like a magnetic force the cake or cookies draw you to where they're stored.

While sweets might appear occasionally, they shouldn't be making regular appearances at your house. Same goes for ice cream, candy, chips, crackers, sugared drinks, and breads that are anything but 100% whole grain.

By far the easiest way to resist temptation is not to face it in the first place. Keep your pantry and fridge stocked with all the real foods I describe in this chapter. When kids (or you) want snacks, get out the carrot sticks, celery, raw peppers, and a few walnuts or peanut or almond butter. Chomp away.

When dessert rolls around, slice an apple and a small piece of good cheese. Just keep the magnetic junk at bay.

Make your daily eating plant-based, with protein

Choosing to eat a plant-based diet most of the time — vegetables, fruits, beans, whole grains, nuts, with meat in any form as a side dish — will unequivocally improve your health in a couple ways. First, these foods are nutrient-dense, meaning there's a powerhouse of nutritional value in the food as it relates to the total number of calories in the food. That's a fancy way of saying you get lots of nutritional bang for your buck.

When you start choosing an apple instead of an apple pastry, a slice of bread made from 100% whole grains over a slice of bread made with refined white or wheat flour, you're beginning to understand the value of eating the food itself instead of something made with a part of that food or a processed version of it.

Focus on increasing the number of fruits and vegetables you eat every day. This can be daunting if you're not in the habit, but the payoff is well worth it. Fruits and veggies contain vitamins, minerals, healthy fats, and roughage in the form of fiber. They strengthen your bones and heart, keep your memory and eyesight sharp, help your blood vessels stay clear, and lower your risk of cancer. Most important, they can help you drop pounds and start your on your way to saying goodbye to fibro.

They're able to do this because they contain phytochemicals

("phyto" means "plant-based"), powerful substances that exist naturally in veggies and fruits as well as in nuts and whole grains. Phytochemicals prevent disease and boost your immune system. Scientists have identified hundreds of phytochemicals in whole foods, and they expect to find many more. Most fruits and vegetables appear to contain more than one kind. All-stars like kale and broccoli have five different types each.

In fact, phytochemicals give fruits and vegetables their colors, so a good rule of thumb is to include as many colors as you can in your daily eating. This idea will lead you naturally to enjoying the widest possible array of produce. In other words, broccoli's great, but if you ate only broccoli you'd be missing the equally powerful—but different—phytochemicals in eggplant, radishes, and sweet potatoes.

Like Eve at the start of this chapter, you might choose to tackle this project with little more than a sharp knife, cutting up raw vegetables and fruits every day to eat when you get hungry, and a basic cookbook that shows you how to prepare good old-fashioned food.

Here's a fact that should please you: once you start cutting out packaged and processed junk foods, instead of taking in all manner of marginal fats and chemicals you'll be able to add your own spices and beneficial fats (no chemicals!), including wonderfully flavored cheeses, olive oil, and avocados. For example, a sweet potato baked and topped with a dollop of sour cream and a sprinkle of cinnamon is a delicious and nutritionally powerful part of lunch or dinner—it's loaded with the phytochemical beta-carotene and also complex carbohydrates to keep your serotonin high.

An avocado (lusciously satisfying and bearing beneficial

fats) sliced into a salad with a fresh tomato, some baby spinach, a hard-boiled egg, and an olive oil dressing provides enough protein and complex carbs to keep your serotonin up, a massive infusion of nutrients, and makes a healthful breakfast, lunch, or dinner. Salad for breakfast? Why not!

Why you should get a vegetable steamer

Here's a key kitchen implement: the vegetable steamer. Nothing fancy—just get yourself one of those round stainless steel collapsible devices with holes that sits inside a pot. Put an inch or two of water in the bottom of the pot, drop in your steamer (which opens to accommodate pans of varying sizes), bring the water to a boil, drop in your veggies, and cover.

Steaming leaves more nutrients in food (so more health-giving nutrients reach your cells) than boiling, which leaves lots in the leftover water. Experiment with steaming times. Some highly nutritious vegetables, such as greens (kale, mustard, collards), are quite fragile, requiring just a few minutes in the steamer. Others, like green beans and broccoli, take longer to make them tender and palatable.

Once you've steamed your veggies, add a flavorful topping, such as an olive oil, fresh lemon, caper, and cheese dressing—or simply toss the vegetables with a little intensely flavored cheese. Cheese? You might wonder, "Won't I gain weight?" Not if you're cutting out all the other junk you formerly ate and if you keep your cheese portions small.

Fruit: get 4 to 6 servings a day

Fruit is an easy and nutritious fast food. A skin-on whole

fruit like an apple or pear — or about half a cup of loose fruit like grapes or berries — represents a serving. If you're pressed for time, shop smartly to ensure you've got enough fruit in the house for a week. If it's just you you're shopping for, count out those apples so you've got one for each day of the week and, by the way, shoot for a variety of types, including as many varieties as your store carries (here in the midwest, our autumn farmers market offers as many as 12 different kinds).

To fulfill your daily servings, ensure you've got enough prunes, grapes, citrus, and any other fruit that you like or that's in season.

Enjoy fruit for breakfast and/or for at least one of your snacks (and dessert) every day. It's a fine source of the carbohydrates that keep your serotonin elevated. Variety is the key here, but there are some obvious standbys, including pitted prunes (often marketed as pitted dried plums), which are loaded with potassium, iron, and antioxidants. Eat a few every day for a serving, either on their own or as a satisfying addition to plain yogurt. They're also delicious cut up and sprinkled on oatmeal or paired with a small piece of hard cheese.

Pack an apple and pear and a small chunk of cheese for a snack at work, or tuck some grapes in with a half sandwich for lunch. You're up to four servings of fruit already and we haven't even covered tossing blueberries or pears into your green salad.

Vegetables: get 5 to 6 servings a day, more if you want

Figure this for a serving: a large handful of loose greens like spinach, kale, or lettuce; a cup of raw veggies, a half cup if they're cooked. Start by being crafty, adding nutrient-packed spinach to sandwiches, chopping greens and spinach finely and adding them to eggs, pastas, soups, and meats. Tuna salad gets a nice boost with finely chopped spinach added to the mix, as does slaw, or add chopped onion or red or green pepper to these salads.

Canned diced tomatoes are easy additions to soups and chili. Experiment with broccoli and cauliflower using a vegetable steamer and a variety of different toppings. One of my favorite veggies in a jar is roasted red peppers.

Salads are maybe the easiest way to get your veggies, but take a pass on iceberg lettuce as it's just crunchy water. Starting with a big handful of spinach and an equal amount of dark romaine lettuce, add a half cup each of four more veggies to meet your day's total. Toss it all with a salad dressing you make from a tablespoon or extra virgin olive oil, a teaspoon of Dijon mustard, and a couple dashes of vinegar.

Spices and herbs

Herbs and spices liven up food and many also are helpful in preventing illness and maintaining good health. Do a little research on herbs—fresh or dried—and start sprinkling them liberally into many foods. Used for thousands of years, cinnamon has been found to lower blood sugar and unhealthy LDL cholesterol. Cinnamon helps insulin move sugar out of the bloodstream and into cells, where it's needed for energy, thus lowering blood sugar. As little as a quarter teaspoon twice a day, sprinkled on your fruit, cereal, or in coffee or tea, is effective and delicious.

Turmeric is another ancient star. This golden orange spice is commonly used in curries, but you can sprinkle a teaspoon into chili, eggs, and soups to gain its beneficial effects, which include acting as an antiinflammatory, antibacterial, and cholesterol-lowering agent.

Researchers also shows that cilantro is in the antibacterial business in addition to bringing its characteristic flavor to many cuisines. One of the compounds in cilantro—duodecenal—is nearly twice as powerful in killing Salmonella (a bacterium that can causes food poisoning) as gentamicin, an antibiotic prescribed by doctors to kill Salmonella.

The Mediterranean diet

To close, a few words about the Mediterranean Diet. By the time you've completed Parts 1-5 of this fibro-friendly eating plan, you've covered all the important aspects of the Mediterranean Diet.

Despite the prevalence of diet books, the Mediterranean way of eating remains the healthiest around. Research shows its generous amounts of fruits and veggies, whole grains, nuts, olive oil (as primary source of fat), a little daily red wine, and some fish and poultry prevents all sorts of chronic illness.

The Mediterranean diet covers you against heart attacks and strokes, cancers of all stripes, and Alzheimer's disease. It may even slow the aging process. All that and fixing your fibro too. Eat well!

10

MEDICATIONS FOR FIBRO: HOW THEY WORK AND HOW THEY CAN HELP

In the annals of fibromyalgia history, the year 2007 is memorable, for this was when the Food and Drug Administration (FDA) approved Lyrica (pregabalin), the first-ever prescription drug for fibromyalgia. There's a twisted reason for the importance of this event, though. In my view it wasn't because of the introduction of an otherwise unremarkable drug (less than 50% of users reported benefits), but rather that it signaled the "legitimization" of fibro as a real and treatable condition in the skeptical minds of a majority of US physicians.

As you likely already know, in order for any drug to receive FDA approval its manufacturers must traverse a challenging terrain that includes lengthy testing and safety protocols. This reaches a climax when researchers present their results, which must show (after a designated period of time taking the drug) that the people in the trial both improved and were not endangered by it.

Additionally, patients taking the drug must be compared by researchers to a similar patient group with the same condition who take a placebo—a dummy pill containing no medicine. The clinical trial must be able to show that the medication users received significantly more benefit than the placebo users. In order to prevent any favoritism toward a drug (remember, physician-researchers are paid vast sums to conduct these trials), researchers don't know until the end of the study who was taking the actual medication and who the placebo.

Same goes for the patients themselves, since the power of the placebo effect is significant (for more on this, see "FDA-approved fibro drugs and the placebo effect"on page 210).

The official term for all this is "randomized placebo-controlled double-blind clinical trial," randomized because patients are selected at random to receive medication or placebo, placebo-controlled because there's a group taking a dummy pill, and double-blind because both patient and researcher are "blind" to the knowledge of whether or not the pill contains actual medicine.

Pharmaceutical companies knew there were a great many people with fibro and each wanted to be first to establish in physician minds the link between fibromyalgia and their drug.

Though first with its fibro drug Lyrica, Pfizer's FDA approval process did not go smoothly. Many physicians on the FDA review panel understood that fibro was not a disease per se, but rather a physical response to chronic stress. They also knew that non-drug therapies like stress reduction, cognitive behavioral therapy, exercise, and massage were quite effective. In short, they were reluctant to "medicalize" fibro for the financial benefit of the pharmaceutical industry. There were also serious concerns about Lyrica's side effects (dizziness, mental confusion, weight gain), the weight gain especially because most fibro patients were overweight already.

Despite these reservations, the FDA did approve Lyrica, and

Pfizer started on the major project of educating both physicians and the public about fibromyalgia. For the next three years, it was a challenge to avoid a TV program or open a magazine without seeing a Lyrica advertisement.

Physician resistance

What would surprise Pfizer, as would later surprise the two other pharmaceutical companies with competing fibro drugs, was the degree of physician resistance to the new drugs. As one pharmaceutical representative said to me, "We expected sales to soar. Our research showed vast numbers of fibromyalgia patients and we thought doctors would say 'Finally, an FDA drug for fibromyalgia!' but it's been an uphill effort."

The reason for this resistance soon became clear. Because most doctors didn't believe fibro existed (no positive test results, remember?), they simply hadn't made any diagnoses of fibromyalgia in their practices. Sure, there were plenty of patients who ached or who were tired all the time, but with fibro low on their diagnostic radar screens the doctors hadn't been connecting the dots. As a result, the drug reps kept hearing "We don't have any fibromyalgia patients," or "I'm reluctant to write a prescription for a condition that's not a disease." Ironically, the reps had been attending lectures on fibro and had learned that 5% to 8% of women had it. Yet they'd walk into a crowded medical office and hear, "We don't have any fibro patients."

But then, as two more fibro medications received FDA approval and the companies began bombarding physicians with informational literature, CDs, dinner conferences, and the like, the tide slowly shifted. More and more physicians began to believe fibromyalgia actually existed (even though too many today still don't).

Unfortunately, and I speak as a physician hired by one of these pharmaceutical companies to lecture doctors about fibro, the vast majority of physicians still don't ask the questions necessary to diagnose fibro in their patients. Nor do they know how to perform a competent physical examination to confirm the diagnosis. (Oddly, their main issue seems to be "What is a 'positive' tender point?" How much fingertip pressure is 4.4 kg? If you press too lightly, you miss a tender point. If too hard, it hurts anyone, with or without fibro.)

Fortunately, the American College of Rheumatology is rethinking its diagnostic guidelines for physicians, broadening them to emphasize the patient's medical history and other symptoms of the fibro spectrum (like depression, headache, and IBS) and de-emphasizing the problematic tender-point diagnosis. Also, the pharmaceutical industry is targeting its efforts more toward the 90% as yet undiagnosed patients who feel achy and tired, reminding them to ask their doctors to consider fibro, with the unstated subtext "if your doctor doesn't believe in fibro, find another doctor."

But let's back up a step. What did doctors treating patients with fibro prescribe before the three FDA-approved drugs? Basically, a slew of medications that dealt with fibromyalgia symptoms: muscle relaxants, pain meds, sleep meds, antidepressants, and the like—any of a couple dozen prescription meds that might offer some relief but hadn't received FDA blessing. This is called "off-label" prescribing, and while not remotely illegal would not hold up well in a malpractice case if anything went wrong (like a fatal side effect) or were a patient to lodge a complaint with a professional review organization. Sadly for fibro patients, many physicians were reluctant to prescribe anything off-label, especially for a condition they didn't believe existed in the first place. We'll review these important off-label medications at the end of this chapter.

These years before 2007 were rough on people with fibro. Between most doctors regarding fibro as non-existent and the lack of FDA-approved medications, if fibro patients weren't tired of hearing "I don't know what's wrong with you—your tests are normal," they were equally tired of hearing (from the physician who finally made the diagnosis) "It looks as if you have fibro but there aren't any medications for it."

In this chapter I'll discuss how each of the FDA-approved fibro medications (Lyrica, Cymbalta, and Savella) can potentially help you.

First, though, a quick review of drugs, side-effects, and a brief exploration of the unique pain of fibro and how the three drugs are designed to resolve it.

Fibro drugs and their side effects

All medications for any condition follow the same basic rules. They're made up of chemicals that, after you ingest them, act on your body in a variety of ways before they're inactivated (metabolized) and excreted. Some drug actions are positive (beneficial clinical effects) and some not so good (side effects). Even here there's a range, however. Some side effects are mild and quite tolerable, while others are either intolerable or downright dangerous. A good drug has a fairly prompt positive clinical result and minimal side effects, a bad drug just the reverse.

The immense seven-pound *Physicians' Desk Reference* (PDR)

that you see in most doctors' offices is literally a bound version of the package inserts for every prescription drug in the US. Were you browse it, you might be surprised to find that most of its pages are devoted to side effects. The general public might be quite surprised to know this, but virtually all doctors are well aware that a majority of the hundreds of prescription drugs are disappointing. If these drugs were students, most would be lucky to receive a C grade.

The three fibro medications are, sadly, no exception to this rule. Each can work for some patients, but certainly not all, and each is mired in its own swamp of side effects. While none of the drugs is particularly dangerous, side effects occur with sufficient frequency that doctors often hear "I can't take this drug" from the fibromyalgia patients attempting to use it.

Part of the side-effect problem with fibro drugs specifically stems from a failure of the pharmaceutical companies to generally appreciate that individual patients are biochemically unique, and that *fibro patients in particular are incredibly chemically sensitive.* The recommended starting doses for all three fibro drugs turned out to be far too high for most patients to tolerate. Doctors began reporting back to the drug companies that patients were abandoning the meds in droves.

Happily, this is slowly changing as doctors working with fibro medications start their patients at much lower doses and increase them very slowly, leveling off when the patient reports feeling better even if the recommended dose hasn't been reached. Later in this chapter, I'll provide specific low-dose instructions for you and your doctor.

A second problem with the three fibro drugs is that they simply don't work for many people taking them. The original clinical trials may have shown "25% more relief than placebo," but while this reflects an improvement it's certainly not a dramatic one. An unfortunately large number (almost half!) of people taking these drugs don't feel much of anything.

Who does best on fibro drugs? People whose fibro is mildest—namely, those who've had it for a year or less. Those with longstanding fibro, whose muscles are deeply and chronically contracted, usually need something in addition to the basic fibro medications.

What causes fibro pain?

Scientists and researchers seeking newer and better medicine for fibro pain control first needed to answer the question, "What causes the pain?" You yourself know that fibro pain is completely different from the pain you feel if you burn your finger on the stove or stub your toe in the dark. Let's review the different types of pain and see where fibro fits in.

There are four distinct forms of pain:

- **Nociceptive** This is the pain caused by an injury. Burning your finger, bumping your head, pulling a back muscle. It's easily identifiable because you know where you hurt yourself, though nociceptive pain can also occur internally, such as from a kidney stone. Compare this type of specific pain (doctors call it "well-localized" pain) with the pain of fibro, where you hurt everywhere.

- **Neuropathic** This pain is caused by damage to a nerve or nerves. Two very common sources of neuropathic pain are diabetes and herpes zoster (shingles). Like nociceptive pain, nerve pain is well-localized to the affected area. Because there is no nerve damage in fibro, fibro is *not* neuropathic pain.

- **Inflammatory** Inflammation is your body's safety mechanism for healing. The redness, swelling, and pain that occur around, say, an infected cut on your arm are the body's well-executed inflammatory response, an elegant mechanism designed to kill germs and promote healing. Like the first two types of pain, inflammatory pain is localized to the area affected. You've probably already discovered that fibro is not inflammatory pain because anti-inflammatory medicines like aspirin or ibuprofen are useless in controlling your fibro misery.

Fibromyalgia's pain category is unique. It is...

- **Abnormal pain processing with central pain amplification.** This medical mouthful is a complicated way of saying what I describe in other chapters. With a processing/amplification disorder, you, as a fibro patient, feel pain more than other people. You feel everything *more*. A stubbed toe for me is a painful temporary annoyance. But in you it can trigger a fibro flare, with a miserable day or two to follow. If I attach a blood pressure cuff to your arm and another to my own arm and inflate them equally, you'll feel pain from the tightening cuff much more intensely than I will. If I place a lightly heated piece of metal on your skin, you'll feel pain while I feel mild discomfort.

Two factors cause people with fibro to receive pain messages differently. First, your low serotonin stress buffer fails to protect you. Second, your nervous system amplifies pain signals by releasing excessive amounts of two pain-related brain chemicals (neurotransmitters): glutamate and Substance P (P, of course, for pain).

We all have these pain chemicals in our bodies to permit us to feel pain. When correctly released, in normal amounts, the chemicals are vitally necessary. They work fast, letting you know, for example, to yank your hand out of a fire rather than wait until you smell burning flesh, to leap off the piece of glass your bare foot just landed on.

From what we now know about fibromyalgia, people with fibro have the correct amount of the pain chemicals glutamate and Substance P in their nerves, but when exposed to anything painful they release too much of the stuff. As a result, they feel pain more than others. Also, for people with fibro the pain is further amplified because of an inadequate serotonin stress-buffering system. If you ponder all this for a moment, you'll see for yourself how fibromyalgia medicines might by designed to work, namely (1) by reducing the amount of glutamate and substance P and (2) raising the serotonin stress buffer.

Beyond serotonin, glutamate, and substance P we have yet another neurotransmitter, norepinephrine, that arises from two sources: the brain and adrenal glands. Among its several jobs, norepinephrine can suppress pain, improve mood, and boost energy. Increasing its levels, therefore, would be a good thing. But chronic stress (and remember that pain itself is a stressor) depletes the adrenal glands of norepinephrine just when it's most required. This slow decline in norepinephrine is one of several reasons why untreated fibro pain gets slowly but steadily worse over time.

In other words, as your adrenals become more and more fatigued with stress and pain, your pain-suppressing, mood elevating, energizing norepinephrine becomes depleted. In the words of an old song, "But you left me…just when I needed you most."

If you're having trouble following this, I can sympathize (med students and practicing physicians have trouble too). Go back and read the last few paragraphs a couple of times and you'll begin to see the overall picture. Also remember that fibromyalgia is *not* a disease, but rather your genetic susceptibility to stress being its old unruly self.

With all this in mind, you'll understand the two biochemical strategies/goals chosen by researchers when developing fibro drugs:

- Block the release of excessive amounts of pain-enhancing chemicals (glutamate and substance P). This is how Lyrica works.

- Increase levels of stress-buffering serotonin and pain-reducing norepinephrine. Cymbalta and Savella are examples of this.

Ask Dr E: Can I Cure My Fibro Without Drugs?

Quick answer: maybe. If you've had fibro for a year or less, you have an excellent chance of turning it around with the steps I outline in the Nearly Natural Cure (page 103).

Even if you've had fibro for longer you stand a good chance of success. I encourage my patients to follow their instincts about this. If you want to try the Nearly Natural Cure, go for it! You have nothing to lose.

But please don't feel inadequate or depressed if that approach doesn't dislodge your fibro. You'll find clear direction at the end of that chapter on how to proceed if this happens to you.

The three FDA-approved fibro drugs

Lyrica

Lyrica (pregabalin) was developed as an advance over a similar medication, Neurontin (gabapentin), whose effectiveness as a pain drug was discovered by accident. Both Neurontin and Lyrica were originally developed (and received FDA approval) as medicines for epilepsy seizures. When seizure patients with certain types of pain began to report the meds were giving them relief, researchers started looking at the drugs seriously for pain control.

(By the way, it's is fairly common for drug companies to cash in on unexpected beneficial side effects. Prozac helped PMS and thus was re-branded and re-marketed as Sarafem. People taking the antidepressant Wellbutrin lost interest in their cigarettes, and now doctors prescribe the same med re-branded as Zyban to help people quit smoking.)

Lyrica and Neurontin work by blocking the brain and nervous system's release of glutamate and substance P. With lower levels of these pain modulators coursing through your body, you feel less pain. Both drugs have been effective for nerve damage (neuropathy) pain and are FDA-approved for diabetic neuropathy and shingles pain. Both can also reduce fibro pain, with Lyrica superior to Neurontin in this regard.

Lyrica may be the best-known of the fibro drugs because it's been so heavily advertised to the public. Doctors, too, have been inundated with promotional material. On the plus side, all that marketing has heightened awareness of fibro, for patients and physicians alike. On the downside, because the makers of Savella, Lyrica's major competitor, steadfastly refuse direct-to-consumer advertising, many patients and too many physicians think Lyrica is the only fibro drug in town. In fact just a handful of doctors are familiar enough with how Lyrica and Savella work to use the two in combination.

Clinical studies show that when taking Lyrica, patients get more relief from fibro pain than when taking a placebo (dummy pill). However, nothing comes without a price, and in Lyrica's case side effects are a major issue. Its dollar cost is also considerable, though no higher than any new drug during its first years on the market.

Lyrica side effects

Lyrica's main side effects are dizziness, sleepiness, unsteadiness as you walk (called ataxia), swelling, and numbness and tingling in the feet and legs. I gave myself a sample dose of Lyrica, as I do with all the meds I prescribe, and by following the company's FDA-approved dosing schedule (75 mg twice daily) lost one full day of my life, either asleep or drowsily staggering around my weekend cabin muttering to myself, "What were these people thinking?"

A real problem with all three fibromyalgia medications (Lyrica, Cymbalta, Savella) has occurred with the approved FDA dosing schedule. Each drug has a suggested "starter schedule," starting low and then moving up. Unfortunately, the schedule is simply increased too quickly for most women with fibromyalgia who are well aware of their sensitivity to drugs and chemicals. The result has been a very substantial "I can't take this medication!" and fibromyalgia patients discontinuing potentially helpful treatments during their first week with the new med.

How to dose your Lyrica

When dosed slowly and correctly, there's real hope for you in Lyrica (Savella and Cymbalta, too). You'll achieve correct dosing by starting at a much lower dose than recommended and increasing it far more slowly than the package insert or FDA recommends. Most likely you've had fibro for years—if you'll be patient, extending the ramp-up period from a week to a month, or even two months, you might get some real benefits you'd otherwise miss because you abandoned the medication prematurely.

Let's first look at Pfizer's FDA-approved dosing schedule for Lyrica: Lyrica 75 mg twice a day for a week, increasing to 150 mg twice a day, and later, if needed, to 150 mg three times a day.

Don't bother. Lyrica capsules are available in 25 mg, 50 mg, 75 mg, 100 mg, 150 mg, 200 mg, 225 mg, and 300 mg sizes. You can take advantage of this impressive spectrum of dose sizes (far more than most new medications) by following my s-l-o-w dosing schedule:

- **Week one** Lyrica 25 mg at bedtime for three days, then 50 mg at bedtime for four days. (Common sense tells us if sleepiness is a side effect, taking it at bedtime until your body gets acclimated would be a good idea.)

- **Week two** Lyrica 25 mg in the morning and 50 mg at bedtime for three days, then 50 mg in the morning and 50 mg at bedtime for four days.

In other words, you'll slowly add no more than 25 mg every three days, with the larger dose taken at bedtime. At this rate, it will take a full six weeks to reach the suggested fibromyalgia dose of 150 mg twice a day.

Your doctor can write you two prescriptions. One for 90

capsules of 25-mg Lyrica, the other for 90 capsules of 50-mg. Then, you take charge of your own slow-dose increases.

A few notes:

- Although it will take six weeks to reach 150 mg twice daily, if you get good relief before that, stop increasing and remain at your effective dose.

- If you increase your dose and get waylaid by side effects, return to your last well-tolerated dose and remain there.

- Consider asking your doctor about adding a small dose of Savella or Cymbalta (see below) if you simply can't go higher on Lyrica and aren't getting relief. In the future, if necessary, you may be able to tolerate a higher dose of Lyrica.

One additional issue with Lyrica is the potential for weight gain. But don't panic.

Once you're past the potential side-effect hurdles with your low-dosing schedule, stay aware of the weight-gain possibility, eat more fresh whole foods, vastly reduce or eliminate sugar and other high-glycemic carbs, and ramp up exercise. These steps themselves will help your fibro. There's much more on all this in the Fibro-Friendly Eating Plan (page 145).

Ask Dr E: Can Lyrica + Savella or Cymbalta be used together?

The short answer is yes.

For the longer answer, understand that Savella and Cymbalta are essentially the same drug, both raising serotonin and norepinephrine. By doing so, fibro pain is diminished and energy increased. Lyrica, on the other hand, helps pain by lowering the pain chemicals glutamate and substance P.

Used together—Lyrica plus either Savella or Cymbalta—you cover all your bases, pain-wise.

Two addition benefits:

- Often, lower doses of the meds are required, so the chances of having side effects is less.

- Some preliminary research is showing that when used in a combination like this, the drugs seem to cancel out each other's side effects.

Cymbalta and Savella

I'll discuss these two together because they have a similar method of action in your body and also carry similar positive and negative side effects.

Both drugs began as antidepressants, Cymbalta (duloxetine) in the US, Savella (milnacipran) in Europe. Their utility for fibro was discovered pretty much by accident, a positive and unexpected side effect that could be turned to financial benefit, the great motivator for pharmaceutical companies.

Most conventional antidepressants are in the SSRI category, including such well known names as Prozac, Celexa, Lexapro, Zoloft, Luvox, and their generics. Many (an astonishing 10% of the US population) people take these for what are called mood disorders—depression, anxiety with panic, obsessive thinking, compulsive behavior, phobias, and so forth. Generally patients do get relief from their symptoms using SSRIs and patient approval ratings on this class of medications is quite high.

SSRI stands for Selective Serotonin Reuptake Inhibitors. These drugs act by increasing brain levels of stress-buffering serotonin. (The herb St. John's wort is a mild but effective SSRI you can try first. It's explained in more detail in the Nearly Natural Cure (page 103).

Here's how SSRIs work: Let's say you're extremely anxious, so much so that you fear leaving your house, and you're plagued by repetitive thoughts about some worst-case scenario. You've been prescribed the SSRI Lexapro, and somewhat nervously you take it. (All patients are nervous swallowing their first prescription drug, by the way). Nothing happens initially, but then, three or four weeks later you realize you're no longer anxious and whatever was obsessing you you now view with calm detachment. People remark that their mood seems much better. You can resume your life.

What you've experienced is your stress buffer going up. You're more protected and resilient. In addition, because of this buffering effect, some, but not all fibro patients taking SSRIs feel their fibro improve, their muscles less tense and painful. But the pharmaceutical industry never got FDA approval for fibromyalgia using its SSRIs because they had better meds in the pipeline.

Both Cymbalta and Savella increase serotonin as well as a second neurotransmitter, norepinephrine, a two-for-the-price-of-one effect. They're thus are classified as SNRIs (serotonin-norepinephrine reuptake inhibitors). The sensible advantage of increasing norepinephrine is its positive effect on mood and energy and a moderate improvement in pain (especially the central pain processing abnormalities of fibro).

Cymbalta had existed in the US for a couple of years as an

antidepressant before getting FDA approval for fibro, and recently received FDA approval for chronic pain in general. The Savella people chose to apply to the FDA solely as a medication for fibro.

Unsurprisingly, the results of the clinical trials for Cymbalta and Savella were similar. With each, about half of patients reported some improvement (the other half did not), including pain reduction, positive mood, better energy, and overall improvement in quality of life.

These positive results are very similar to Lyrica. In other words, despite the cheery looking woman in the TV ads who acts like her fibro is gone and now she's returning to the daily grind we know as life, she's got a 50-50 chance of success with Lyrica as well as Cymbalta and Savella. There have been no published clinical trials using the combination of Lyrica PLUS either Cymbalta or Savella, but fibromyalgia specialists prescribing two together have reported definite benefits.

Cymbalta and Savella side effects

Because Cymbalta and Savella act similarly, their side effects are virtually identical. The single most "I can't take this" side effect is nausea, with patients nicknaming Cymbalta "Cymbarfta." This nausea occurs, as do headache, palpitations, insomnia, and sweating, because of rising norepinephrine levels, which is what the drug is supposed to do. However, if the norepinephrine rise is slowed down by gradually increasing the dose, side effects are dramatically lessened.

Unfortunately, just like with Lyrica, the manufacturers of Cymbalta and Savella failed to take into account the chemical sensitivity of people with fibro. Both manufacturers recommend increasing the dose to the FDA-approved level over the span of a single week, reaching the target dose in seven days. For people with fibro, this is too much norepinephrine too soon. Doctors prescribing these drugs began getting frantic callbacks from patients disappointed that they were unable to tolerate a medication that might have given them relief.

How to dose your Cymbalta or Savella

Cymbalta comes in capsules of 20 mg, 30 mg, and 60 mg. The suggested fibro maintenance dose of 60 mg daily is designed to be reached after one week of 30-mg capsules. Men, with higher levels of serotonin, can generally handle this. Women barf.

When I prescribe Cymbalta, I recommend the following schedule:

Weeks 1 and 2 – 20 mg daily in the morning
Weeks 3 and 4 – 30 mg daily in the morning
Weeks 5 and 6 – 40 mg (two 20-mg capsules daily in the morning)
Thereafter 60 mg (one 60-mg capsule daily in the morning (as maintenance)

Ask your doctor for:

- 42 capsules of Cymbalta 20 mg (for weeks 1, 2, 5 and 6)
- 14 capsules of Cymbalta 30 mg (for weeks 3 and 4)
- 30 capsules of Cymbalta 60 mg (as maintenance)

DO NOT FILL ALL THREE PRESCRIPTIONS THE SAME DAY. Your insurance will "deny." Fill each prescription the day before you need to start it.

Savella comes in tablet form: 12.5 mg, 25 mg, 50 mg, and 100 mg. The most common successful dose during clinical trials was 50 mg twice daily.

Savella's maker, Forest Labs, suggests one day of 12.5 mg at bedtime, 12.5 mg twice daily for two more days, 25 mg twice daily for four days, and then at day eight you're on the maintenance dose of 50 mg twice daily. They provided doctors with a "starter pack" that looked like a card of birth control pills. Most of my patients on this dosing schedule were really nauseated after a week and unable to even think about increasing to 50 mg twice daily.

And yet Savella works in low doses. You just have to be patient.

When I prescribe Savella, I recommend this schedule:

Week 1 – 12.5 mg at bedtime for four days (if you're especially sensitive, 6.25 mg—half a tablet), increasing to 12.5 mg twice a day for three days.
Week 2 12.5 mg in the morning and 25 mg in the evening for the full week.
Week 3 25 mg twice daily (some patients get good results at this dose and can maintain themselves here).
Week 4 25 mg in the morning and 37.5 mg (one 25 mg + one 12.5 mg) at bedtime.
Week 5 37.5 mg twice daily.
Week 6 37.5 mg in morning, 50 mg at bedtime.
Week 7 and thereafter 50 mg twice daily.

Ask your doctor for:

- 45 tablets of Savella 12.5 mg (for weeks 1, 2, 5 and 6)
- 60 tablets of Savella 25 mg (for weeks 2, 3, 4, and 5)
- 60 tablets of Savella 50 mg (as maintenance)

DO NOT FILL ALL THREE PRESCRIPTIONS THE SAME DAY. Your insurance will "deny." Fill each prescription the day before you need to start it. Also, most insurance companies only allow 60 tablets at a time, so you might need to refill your 25-mg size.

My low-dose schedules have dramatically reduced the number of e-mails I receive from patients saying, "I can't take this. I am so nauseated."

Overall, I'd estimate at least one third of my fibro patients do well enough on the lower, ramp-up period doses that they don't need to increase to the maximum. And, of course, by keeping the doses low and the ramp-up s-l-o-w, the risk of side effects is much lower than at the full "approved" dose.

Patients are guardedly happy with the new fibromyalgia medications. "Guardedly" because although the drugs get at the pain and improve energy, despite best intentions, side effects can start appearing any time and patients are confronted with the big decision, "Is it worth it?" You, personally, may be delighted or disappointed, and there's no way to predict your personal response except to give it a try.

Of the three FDA-approved fibro drugs, my preference

Overall, all three medications get a "C" grade from me, but currently they're what we've got to work with. My average grade is driven by the fact that each has a roughly 50% chance of working...plus all those side effects. Compare fibro meds to blood pressure drugs and the difference is clear. For high blood pressure, you can easily find a grade-A, nearly side-effect free medication that works effectively most of the time.

Of the three fibro drugs, my guarded preference has been for Savella for several reasons. Full disclosure: I was hired by Forest Labs, makers of Savella, to give educational lectures to doctors about fibro. Why did I, a frequent online critic of pharmaceutical companies, take the job? Because it was chance to enlighten physicians on fibro and give them the benefit of what I've learned in my 20 years of treating it.

Here's why I slightly prefer Savella:

- Although I'm puzzled by the promotional literature accompanying Savella and Cymbalta because of the sentence "The exact mechanism of how (Savella/Cymbalta) inhibits central pain is unknown," this must have been an obscure FDA requirement. We do know how these meds work. Raising serotonin improves a person's stress-buffering system and allows tensed muscles to relax. Raising norepinephrine improves energy and mood while reducing response to pain. To me, these drugs come as close as anything to correcting fibro's underlying neurotransmitter issues: low serotonin and low norepinephrine.

- Lyrica is essentially a pain medication that happens to work for some people with fibro. It does not correct fibro's serotonin/norepinephrine imbalances. I limit my prescribing of Lyrica as an occasional add-on to Savella and suggest you do the same.

- For unclear reasons, Cymbalta seems to lose its mojo after about a year. My patients and I usually try increasing the Cymbalta dose at that point, but after a few months we're compelled to try something else.

- I like that Savella is available in a lower dose than either of the others. This means you can start taking Savella at a 12.5-mg dose (a mere 12.5% of the 100-mg per day maintenance dose) or even lower by breaking and taking half a tablet. Cymbalta and Lyrica come in capsule form, making the half-pill impossible. Cymbalta's lowest starting dose is 20 mg (33% of the 60-mg maintenance dose—far higher than Savella).

Ask Dr E: My doctor has me on Cymbalta and I think it's working. Will I have to take it forever?

In all likelihood, no. Once you've broken the stress>pain>more stress>more pain cycle by raising your serotonin and norepinephrine plus maintaining your well-being by following the steps in the Nearly Natural Cure, you can discuss with your doctor tapering and eventually discontinuing the Cymbalta.

Which patients can benefit from these fibro meds?

Just about now, you might be mumbling to yourself, "I thought Dr E was a more natural doctor, using herbs and alternative treatments. This reads like a chemistry book." Before you toss this precious book into the fire, let me summarize who can benefit from the FDA-approved fibro drugs...and why.

With 12 million people with fibro in the US, you'd expect that patients fall at varying points on the fibro continuum ranging from pretty mild to awful and disabling. And that's exactly what we have.

- **If you have mild to moderate fibro**, you don't necessarily need medication unless you choose to try it.

Our clinic is a patient-directed practice, meaning we encourage patients to seek treatment paths they feel most comfortable using. If you're a person who estimates her fibro started roughly a year ago or less (with some days both good and bad) and you came to our clinic we'd recommend a blend of non-pharmacologic treatments, including nutritional supplements, diet changes, myofascial release therapy or chiropractic, acupuncture, a slow but steadily increasing exercise program, and perhaps counseling. I walk you through this plan in detail in the Nearly Natural Cure (page 103). In addition, if needed, we might prescribe thyroid hormone replacement or adrenal hormone replacement if your tests showed thyroid or adrenal fatigue. We'd also prescribe pain medication if needed for bad days — what's called "breakthrough pain."

- **If you have fibro that ranges from moderate to severely disabling** you most likely do need prescription medication (namely, one of the three FDA-approved drugs) to break the pain-stress-pain cycle. In addition, we'd encourage you to do everything listed in the paragraph just above and you'll possibly need one or more of the off-label medications described in the following section.

The treatment goal for any person with fibro? To effectively break that cycle of pain-stress-pain. And then, to trim as many medications as possible from your regimen. Some people with fibro are able to walk away from all medications. Others need a permanent supplement for serotonin support, a maintenance sleeping pill, a muscle relaxant, and/or even a pain pill for a sudden and unexpected fibro flare.

No two of you are alike. And thus there is no single solution.

FDA-approved fibro drugs and the placebo effect

The term placebo comes from the Latin, "I shall please." For a doctor to give a patient a placebo means she's dispensing a substance that has no known beneficial effect. That's because placebos contain no actual medicine.

Treating patients with what's essentially deliberate deception has generated a lot of controversy among physicians around the world. American doctors were recently shocked to learn that 50% of the prescriptions written by physicians in Germany were placebos, and that the German Medical Association (GMA) encouraged doctors to use placebos at an even higher rate. The GMA's stance was that the power of the mind and the power of suggestion had such profound effects on healing and symptom relief that physicians should tap into it, rather than endlessly prescribing drugs of dubious merit and potential harm.

The human response to placebos has a lot to teach us about the power of our minds. In recent studies, PET scans taken of the brains of actively meditating people revealed that the areas involved in pain perception actually appeared to calm down during meditation…simultaneously with the meditator herself reporting less and less pain. The effect carried forward too. Weeks later, with continued regular meditation, patients reported dramatic reductions in their overall pain levels. In other words, whether you're practicing regular meditation or your mind is being "fooled" by taking a placebo, consciously or unconsciously you are tapping into the power of your mind to lessen fibromyalgia pain.

Let's review the math on the clinical trials of the FDA-approved fibro medications vs the power of the placebo.

During the trials of all three drugs, approximately 45% of those taking actual medication reported benefits, while 22% of those taking a placebo reported equally good benefits. This difference—medication performing twice as well as placebo—is considered by the FDA to be sufficient evidence to warrant approving a drug as being effective. Obviously if both drug and placebo came back equally effective the drug would receive a thumbs-down.

But the 22% of women in the study—that's almost a quarter of the total—because they were given a placebo were *unconsciously* using the power of their minds to get pain relief.

Since it's unlikely you'll ever be in a fibromyalgia drug clinical trial and because US physicians virtually never deliberately prescribe placebos, with guided meditation (find details in the Nearly Natural Cure) you can *consciously* use your mind power on your fibromyalgia.

This isn't to suggest in any way that your fibro is "all in your head," but rather that when you understand your body, are no longer frightened by what you're experiencing, and feel reasonably confident you can get control of your fibro, your symptoms will lessen before you swallow your very first pill (if pill-swallowing is part of your fibro treatment).

One final point about clinical trials that's worth pondering: volunteers for these studies are paid and want to please the researcher so they'll be asked back to be in other studies. With a dramatic side effect like nausea or dizziness, volunteers immediately know they're taking an actual drug and many unconsciously exaggerate the drug's benefits.

Drug studies are never performed using placebos that cause harmless side effects (called "active placebos") because both groups would then be trying to please the researcher, in which case the difference between the drug and placebo might turn out to be unimpressive and inadequate to earn FDA approval.

Other helpful fibro medicines

Before the release of the FDA-approved fibro drugs, conventional medical treatment was hit or miss. I do like the "Whack-A-Mole" analogy, as you've noted. This carnival game features a plastic mole that pops up and when you knock it down with your mallet, up pop two more. With fibro, the moles are symptoms.

(With no false modesty, I am actually very good at this game and, if available, will play with not one mallet but two, my hands flying across the game board, lights flashing, bells ringing. If asked how I managed to become this skilled at this particular game, I lower my voice an octave in an attempt to sound exactly like Harrison Ford as Indiana Jones and reply, "I treat fibromyalgia.")

Here is Whack-A-Mole treatment for fibro: "My muscles are so tight, and they ache," you might have said to your doctor before the FDA fibro drugs were available. In response, your physician may have prescribed a muscle relaxant and, if you were fortunate, a pain med. "And I'm not sleeping..." So then came a sleep med prescription. Doctors then discovered, pretty much by accident, that certain antidepressants helped their fibro patients and that a medicine designed for daytime sleepiness gave patients a decent energy boost.

Little by little, you saw your countertop filling with all these drugs and you may have wondered: Will I ever be able to get off them? (The answer is yes, and more on this below.)

All this defines one of the central problems with conventional medicine. When the only tool in your doc's toolbox is a prescription pad, you can expect to receive prescriptions. Sadly, most well-meaning doctors never reach out to fibro-effective alternative therapists like acupuncturists, chiropractors, and myofascial release therapists, even though each of these practitioners can absolutely reduce your reliance on drugs. Very few fibro patients are ever referred for a form of psychotherapy called cognitive behavioral therapy, which has been repeatedly shown to be beneficial.

So great is the reliance on pharmaceuticals that in a published survey of fibro patients, all were taking at least two prescription meds and almost 25% were taking *five or more separate drugs every day, each drug* with its own goodie bag of side effects, a fact I don't need to remind you about.

While the FDA-approved fibro meds Lyrica, Savella, and Cymbalta have reduced the need for so many individual medications, they're far from perfect. Even their manufacturers acknowledge the drugs are effective for less than half the people who take them. Side effects range from annoying to deal-breaking, with only the rare patient ever saying "My fibro is gone and I had no side effects."

My message in this section? Despite the newer fibro-specific drugs, many of you will want to consider how adding other medications can help. Before I get into the specifics, let me reiterate my treatment objectives for the fibro patients we see at our clinic.

Generally, a combination of prescription medications,

nutritional therapies, and alternative practitioners is required. I try to use as few prescription drugs as possible, but I eschew the type of ideological thinking that maintains "I don't believe in any drugs for fibro" because this approach can obstruct your chances for a happy, healthy, and fulfilled life. Each patient is completely unique. Some can move forward with nutritional supplements and bodywork therapies alone, others need prescription medications. For any practitioner, MD or otherwise, to approach all fibro patients with a "no medications under any circumstances" forces that practitioner's ideology at the peril of his patient's well-being.

My fibro treatment objectives are…

Pain reduction On a scale of 1 to10, with 10 being severe daily pain, reduce pain to a tolerable 1 or 2, anticipating episodes of worsening pain, called fibro flares, from unexpected stresses (bad week at work, change in weather, etc).

1. **Improved sleep** A decent night's sleep and waking up feeling refreshed.

2. **Energy** Sufficient day-to-day energy to uninterruptedly continue your responsibilities for career, home, relationship, children — whatever's central to your life.

3. **Mood** A generally positive mental attitude despite the challenge of getting symptoms under control.

4. **Focus and concentration skills** We want to see good control here.

5. **Medication reduction** Ultimately, as fibro symptoms recede, begin a slow reduction of all medications. And ideally at some point you'll be able to refer to the time

"When I had fibro."

I've organized these additional fibro medications based on symptoms so you can easily review options according to what ails you. Not one of these drugs was developed specifically for fibro. Rather, they gained their reputation via the hit-or-miss technique doctors use when confronted with symptoms (from any condition) that defy common explanation. Pain control gets its own chapter, (page 227) because using potent pain medications for fibro is still considered controversial by some physicians, though not at all by me.

Off-label prescribing

Let's quickly review the meaning of the term "off-label prescribing." Virtually all prescription drugs are officially approved by the Food and Drug Administration (FDA), an immense bureaucracy that regulates the vast segment of our economy that the words "food" and "drugs" imply. (Though somehow the FDA still can't seem to get cigarettes off the market). Before any drug is available for prescription, it must pass muster with a series of clinical trials and then meet the approval of several separate FDA committees.

When a drug is finally approved, this approval applies only to the drug being used for a specific medical condition. Drug A is approved for diabetes, Drug B for migraine, and so forth. Even if Drug B, the migraine drug, is later found to help diabetes, the manufacturer cannot reveal this information to physicians without re-initiating the entire FDA approval process and performing clinical trials that prove Drug B is effective for the new condition.

And while it's not remotely illegal for a doctor to prescribe off-label, many physicians, fearing a visit from a malpractice attorney, prescribe strictly according to FDA approval guidelines.

So, assume medicine for disease A is found to be really helpful for disease B. If a doctor goes ahead and writes the prescription, she is prescribing off-label, and there's much precedent for doing so. When the blood pressure meds called beta-blockers were found to be excellent at preventing migraines, it took a decade of off-label prescribing (and, eventually, the required clinical trials) to add migraine prevention to the FDA's approved-use list for beta blockers.

If a new use for an older drug is uncovered, the pharmaceutical companies themselves are forbidden to breathe a word about it to physicians or the public until the clinical trials are completed. When physicians reported the epilepsy drug Neurontin helped some of their patients with fibro, drug reps from Neurontin's manufacturer Pfizer Labs began spreading the word, with the result that the company was fined $430 million for illegal marketing, even though the drug benefitted some patients. These days, a drug rep would sooner cut off her tongue than discuss an off-label use of the drug she's touting.

Because not one of the drugs below is actually FDA-approved for fibro, vast numbers of people have been denied medications that might have offered some relief, partly because physicians fear the largely imaginary consequences off-label prescribing.

The first antidepressants
The first antidepressants got their start as fibro medications by an odd route. Before anyone understood anything about fibro—before it was actually named as a real condition—women were showing up in doctors' offices, and later

rheumatology clinics, with widespread muscle pain, fatigue, and negative test results. With mostly minimal physician empathy ("She's back again, always complaining..."), in the 1960s and 1970s this group of women was written off as being depressed and was either referred for psychiatric help or prescribed one of the then newly released antidepressants.

Because the SSRI antidepressants such as Prozac and Zoloft wouldn't be developed for a few years, the prescription was for one of the tricyclic antidepressants—Elavil (amitriptyline) or Pamelor (nortriptyline)—or a related tetracyclic antidepressant such as Desyrel (trazodone).

After a few weeks, when her symptoms started improving, you can imagine one of these patients scratching her head in wonderment, thinking, "The doctor must have been right. Maybe I *was* depressed." We now know a bit more about what these first antidepressants were actually doing and, I might add, what they continue to do as part of the fibro armamentarium.

1. The early antidepressants act by raising both serotonin (stress buffer) and norepinephrine (mood, energy, natural pain control). By a different mechanism of action they're essentially a primitive form of Savella or Cymbalta.

2. They also work similarly to the muscle relaxant cyclobenzaprine (Flexeril—more on this below).

3. The major side effect of all three, drowsiness, was the main reason people disliked them. However, when taken at bedtime they induced deep and reasonably efficient sleep. As any fibro patient knows, pain and energy are greatly improved after deep and refreshing sleep.

Thus, sleeping better, with muscles relaxing at night and rising levels of stress-buffering serotonin and pain-killing norepinephrine, many people taking these drugs for fibro did indeed feel better, and to this day these meds continue to help many people with fibromyalgia. But not because they were "depressed all along."

SSRI antidepressants

The SSRIs (selective serotonin reuptake inhibitors) were introduced in 1987 with the release of Prozac. The SSRIs now includes Zoloft, Celexa, Lexapro, and Paxil as well as SNRIs (serotonin and norepinephrine reuptake inhibitors) such as Effexor, Pristiq, and Cymbalta. (Savella is also in the SNRI class, but while it was originally marketed as an antidepressant in Europe its manufacturer limited its US FDA application for fibro.)

Although fibro had become better known, physicians persisted in their belief that women who had it were "just depressed," and prescribed an SSRI, with mildly positive results. Pharmacologically speaking, you'd expect this when you consider SSRIs do raise the serotonin stress-buffering system, allowing a woman with fibro to stop tensing her muscles against a hostile world.

But then doctors began to appreciate that the even newer group of antidepressants, the SNRIs (because they boosted both serotonin and norepinephrine), worked better against fibro than any of the SSRIs. The first SNRI was venlafaxine (Effexor), and it worked fairly well. It was followed a few years later by duloxetine (Cymbalta), which proved more effective. The difference, it turned out, lay in the norepinephrine effect. Cymbalta raised norepinephrine more efficiently than Effexor. The key for fibro is raising both serotonin and norepinephrine, and the more norepinephrine the better. (Read about the SNRIs Cymbalta and Savella on page 201 for a more complete explanation.)

Today, most physicians treating people with fibro do not prescribe SSRIs to control fibro pain, but rather one of the SNRIs. For the many fibro patients who are already taking an SSRI for depression or anxiety, generally the SNRI can be safely added. The so-called serotonin syndrome (two meds having the effect of creating too much serotonin) is much more written about than actually ever seen.

The real problem with both the SSRIs and the SNRIs are their side effects, which for SSRIs include sexual dysfunction (sex drive and orgasm become distant memories for many users), weight gain, and feeling emotionally numb. The latter is caused by your rising serotonin pushing you into the levels men have — welcome to Guyville.

SNRI side effects are nausea as your norepinephrine rises and hot flashes/excessive sweating/palpitations (again from the norepinephrine effect), though they cause less sexual dysfunction and weight gain than the SSRIs.

To see how nutritional supplements can be used to achieve similar results without the side effects, read the Nearly Natural Cure (page 103). You'll note I recommend St. John's wort, which acts as a mild SSRI (raising serotonin), the amino acid 5HTP (5 hydroxytryptophan), which acts like a tricyclic antidepressant (also raising serotonin), and the amino acid DL Phenylalanine, which boosts norepinephrine.

Muscle relaxants

It was likely an act of desperation on the part of physicians to prescribe muscle relaxants for fibro. Here were patients describing chronic muscle tension and pain and these were medicines that relaxed muscles. Seemed like a good fit.

Unfortunately, with the exception of cyclobenzaprine (Flexeril), muscle relaxants have disappointing results. One problem is that their muscle-relaxing effect is only temporary and not for the long-term needs of fibro. It was with good reason these drugs were FDA-approved for "acute muscle spasm" — such as when you pull your back or strain your neck. In addition, for most people the side effects are unacceptable: drowsiness and dry mouth.

Cyclobenzaprine (Flexeril) is widely prescribed off-label for fibro because its effect is very similar to the early tricyclic antidepressant amitriptyline (Elavil). It increases your serotonin stress buffer and makes you so sleepy you can use it as a sleep med. To avoid next-day drowsiness, I suggest patients begin with a half tablet (5 mg), taking it no later than 9:30 pm. With that schedule, the drowsiness effect has pretty much worn off by the next morning. Unfortunately for some women, the side effects linger no matter when the med is taken and Flexeril becomes unacceptable.

One of the more exciting developments in off-label fibro treatment is a newer time-release form of cyclobenzaprine (Amrix). While Flexeril and other muscle relaxants work for just three or four hours, Amrix provides muscle relaxation for a full 24 hours. At this point, it's not FDA-approved for fibro and, fearing FDA fines, Amrix drug reps will not discuss its use for fibro with doctors. But you can ask your doctor to prescribe it.

When I wrote the manufacturer about prescribing Amrix for fibro, I received a curt form letter asking me to limit my prescribing of Amrix to its FDA-approved use: short-term muscle spasm. They didn't confirm or deny they were conducting clinical trials using Amrix for fibro, though I know one is currently underway. That $430 million fine against Pfizer would bankrupt the Amrix manufacturer, so I can appreciate their being tight-lipped about this.

Sleep medications

People with fibro pray for a decent night's sleep. Many report not having slept well for years. How could you possibly sleep when every time you get remotely comfortable, something hurts because you're lying on a fibro tender point? So you shift in bed to relieve the pain, but soon it returns in a new location. To make matters worse, lying there, your muscles tense and stiffen further. Even shifting positions hurts. When finally it's morning, you attempt to climb out of bed and you feel like a Mack truck ran over you during the night. Your partner jumps out of bed and heads briskly to the bathroom, the kids are racing through the house, and everyone wants something from you. But you're exhausted, everything hurts, and you move slowly and painfully, like the rusty tin man in the Wizard of Oz.

After a deep sleep, however, your world is completely different. Yes, you're still a bit stiff, but somehow better: less pain, more energy, better mood. Ah, if only.

I once heard a lecturer on fibro tell his physician audience, "If you can help a fibro patient sleep deeply every single night, you'll be halfway to solving her fibro." I believe this. Virtually all doctors who regularly treat people with fibro are aware that a profound sleep disorder lies at the heart of fibro.

If you need a maintenance sleep med every single night for the rest of your incarnation (you'll be better in your next life) to keep your fibro at bay, then so be it. Decent, refreshing sleep is vital to your well-being.

One of my patients burst into grateful tears when I told her it was okay to use a sleep med every night and to forget about feeling guilty for doing so. It was the only way she felt reasonably well during the day. Her previous doctor, bless his soul, told her she was heading down the road to drug addiction and an early death. Every single time she swallowed a sleeping pill, she felt a tsunami of guilt. I said, "Forget it and take the sleep med."

Instead of prescribing a sleep medication, many fibro doctors instead prescribe one of the early antidepressants (Trazodone, Elavil, etc., see page 216) because they make you very sleepy, raise your serotonin, and act similarly to Flexeril as a muscle relaxant. Other doctors prescribe Flexeril as a sleep med for the same three reasons. Whatever works for you is just fine with me.

There are just a handful of sleep meds that actually work

Here they are:

- Ambien (zolpidem, both regular and the long-acting CR version)
- Lunesta (eszopiclone)
- Restoril (temazepam)
- Sonata (zaleplon)

The first three seem equally effective, but my patients do have preferences.

Some feel Sonata is too short-acting, meaning if you take it at 10 pm you wake up feeling pretty energetic at 2 am and can't get back to sleep. For this reason, Sonata is a good medication to use if you fall asleep easily without meds, but awaken in the middle of the night. Take Sonata as late as 2 am and it will be out of your system by 6 am. Take any of the others at that hour and you'll sleep though your alarm clock. The recently introduced sleep drug Rozerem is about as effective as a cup of chamomile tea.

Anti-anxiety drugs for sleep

To encourage sleep, some physicians add (or substitute) an anti-anxiety medication such as alprazolam (Xanax), clonazepam (Klonopin), or lorazepam (Ativan).

The problem here is that since these are not sleep meds, patients tend to self-increase their dose in order to fall asleep. As they do so, their brains become more and more dependent on the drug and if they stop taking it suddenly (like leaving the bottle at home when on vacation), they go into actual withdrawal symptoms, including seizures.

This virtually never occurs if the dose remains steady and is *not* increased without your physician's OK.

A note about Xyrem for sleep

It's worth mentioning one final sleep med you may have heard about, though it's unlikely your doctor will ever prescribe it (and just as unlikely your insurance company will pay for it). Xyrem (sodium oxybate) might well be called the "mother of all sleep medications," and as the cost is roughly $4,200 a month it definitely had better be good.

The origin of Xyrem is the infamous date-rape drug gamma hydroxybutyrate (GHB). It induces very deep sleep in a matter of minutes. Physicians who specialize in sleep medicine knew that one of the best treatments for narcolepsy (excessive daytime sleepiness) was to induce deep and efficient sleep during nighttime hours. Xyrem will do just that.

It's a liquid, and to use it you pour two separate doses and prepare yourself for the night. You take the first dose, turn out your light, and you're asleep in minutes. But three hours later, a pillow alarm clock rings (the company supplies this) and you reach over, take the second dose, and return to sleep. Many people don't even remember taking their second dose.

The reason for this strange state of affairs is that Xyrem is metabolized by your body so quickly that unless you take a second dose, you'll awaken at about 2 am but be unable to fall back asleep.

When you have fibro, sleeping deeply will make the following day almost blissful. So fibro doctors began prescribing Xyrem off-label for patients who simply weren't falling asleep with conventional medications like Elavil, Ambien, Lunesta, or Trazodone. The results were impressive enough (good sleep, less fibro pain, better energy) that the company petitioned the FDA to allow further testing in an effort to get approval of Xyrem specifically for fibro.

The clinical trials actually went well, with fibromyalgia patients reporting reduced pain and more energy. However, the FDA voted a unanimous "no!" for fibro use—not because Xyrem wasn't effective, but because of their reasonable concern about making a drug with a high potential for abuse (as in date rape) available by prescription.

There aren't many people with narcolepsy, but there are 12 million with fibro. The idea of thousands of gallons of a date-rape drug literally and figuratively flooding the market was too much risk. Thus Xyrem remains available for narcolepsy only, but you can ask your physician to off-label prescribe it if you've not found sound sleep with other sleep meds. Unless, she's familiar with Xyrem, expect a "no."

Stimulants

There are a variety of medicines designed to make you more alert, to energize you and stimulate your brain. We're most familiar with caffeine, of course, and many of us with fatigue or brain fog (or just because we're addicted to caffeine) head to our local Starbucks to prepare for a work day.

It's true, though, that many fibro patients who have learned to cope with pain sometimes simply cannot manage the fatigue. And while much of a fibro patient's fatigue can be attributed to adrenal and/or thyroid exhaustion, and, as such, can be treated, there will always be some people who remain fatigued no matter what.

When trying to remedy fatigue, doctors first try to deepen sleep, normalize adrenal and thyroid function, and reduce pain. When fatigue persists, many physicians turn to stimulant medications.

The two most commonly used are modafinil (Provigil) and armodafinil (Nuvigil), and again, you must rely on your doctor being willing to prescribe off-label. The only FDA approved use of these medications is for narcolepsy (excessive daytime sleepiness) and shift-work sleep disorder, which is exactly what it sounds like. Just like Xyrem deepens sleep, stimulants wake you up.

How they work is not exactly clear, but likely they increase levels of dopamine, your wake-up neurotransmitter. In this regard, they're similar to the familiar medications for attention deficit disorder—Adderall, Ritalin, Concerta, and Vyvanse. In fact, all four of these are also occasionally prescribed for chronic fatigue syndrome and the severe fatigue of fibro.

Pain
You might think it odd that since fibro is primarily a chronic pain syndrome, I have yet to discuss pain management drugs. These merit their own chapter, and you'll find it on page 227.

Do I need all these meds for fibro?
No. Many of the actions of these various pharmaceuticals can be very closely duplicated by nutritional supplements, Chinese medicine (herbs and acupuncture), psychotherapy (especially cognitive behavioral therapy), and bodywork therapies (like myofascial release).

You might require some medication in the first weeks or months of treating your fibro, but all of them, forever? Again, no.

But now you should clearly see the reasons for the survey showing that fibro patients use multiple medications, that 25% of fibro patients regularly take five or more prescription drugs every day.

Use them as needed, and then wean yourself off them. Work with the Nearly Natural Cure (page 103) to receive the non-drug support that will make your fibro a memory.

11

PAIN DRUGS FOR FIBRO

Warning: Offering adequate pain relief to people with fibro is highly controversial among physicians. This chapter may not be greeted with the approval of many physicians, including possibly your own.

Right now a majority of US physicians stubbornly believe that despite your fibro pain, you shouldn't use pain medicines for relief. That no matter how severe and disabling your pain, you should essentially try anything else—antidepressants, muscle relaxants, epilepsy drugs, sleeping pills, anti-inflammatory medications, energizers—everything except pain medications.

Shocking, isn't it?

When I use the term pain drugs, I mean drugs in the opioid family, the name derived, of course, from opium, which comes from the stunningly beautiful poppy, grown primarily in southern Asia to provide the world with heroin. Thus, even the word "opioid," a classification of many effective pain medications, carries a burden of negative connotation.

Opium, heroin, morphine, addiction, drug wars, rehab, Rush Limbaugh—all enough to frighten people away, patients and doctors alike.

But the opioid issue is argued heatedly among doctors. Last

year, after a fibro meeting, discussing the chronic pelvic pain of fibro, one physician said "I'd rather schedule a hysterectomy than write her a Vicodin prescription."

If I were one of his patients, I'd keep a watchful eye on my uterus.

Letting your imagination run wild, you might envision all sorts of dreadful outcomes of taking something for your pain and decide to simply live with it. But saying no to pain medications when you spend your days in constant pain is the ultimate example of throwing the baby out with the bath water.

I believe the pain medicine fear factor is responsible for our current problem of inadequately treated chronic pain (arising from fibro or any condition). Pain *mismanagement* has its roots in medical school, where young doctors are incorrectly taught that all decent pain drugs should be reserved for short-term use by two groups of patients: people with acute injuries and those who have post-operative pain.

Providing adequate pain relief to a third group, cancer patients, is a relatively recent phenomenon. To this day, many physicians reserve their pain med prescribing to the final weeks or days of a person's life rather than starting it sooner. When my father-in-law was dying of lung cancer a few years ago, I could see he was in pain, and although his doctor had prescribed a small amount of low-strength Vicodin he was reluctant to use it, having been warned by both his physician and pharmacist that he could become addicted to it.

If you can see the scathing irony in that scenario, you understand why this typical example of pain *mismanagement* needs fixing.

Patient Stories: How Laura's Dental Surgery
Led to Fibro Pain Relief

On Laura's first visit she told me she'd had fibro for many years and had always been told by doctors that nothing could be done to help. Her doctor had recommended she try "something safe for the pain" like Tylenol or ibuprofen (neither of which, by the way, could ever be considered safe, due to their potential to cause significant stomach, liver, and kidney problems).

And predictably, neither made a dent in her fibro pain.

I asked Laura if she'd ever found anything that helped her pain. A flash of embarrassment crossed her face.

"Yes, one thing. This..." she said, scrabbling through her purse. "I got these pills from my dentist a couple years ago after some really painful dental work. I took one and for a couple of hours my fibro pain just melted away. It was amazing. I experimented the next day and the same thing happened. So I made an appointment with my doctor and took the pills with me, so I could show him what had made me feel better."

"And?" I prompted...

"He got really angry and told me he'd never, ever prescribe anything like this for fibromyalgia. That it was okay for dental work, but if I used it for fibro I could become a dope addict. He was very upset and I felt ashamed, like some sort of criminal, and then I got angry that he could even think that about me."

"But I see you still have the bottle," I said. "Did you get a refill?"

"No. I have six pills left. I got twelve originally from the dental work and I guess they're kind of old now, but I promised myself I wouldn't use them unless my fibro got really really bad."

The tablets were Vicodin, a combination of hydrocodone and acetaminophen and a favorite of dentists for pain control. Over the years, many of my patients have told me that their fibro pain seemed to vanish during the hours after taking dentist-prescribed Vicodin.

How beautifully Laura's story illustrates the fact that easing the pain can make fibro feel like it's gone. And how clearly it shows where many physicians stand on this issue. And, by the way, Laura did depart that day with a prescription to freshen up her Vicodin.

Advances in the use of pain meds

In recent years, thanks to many pain therapy conferences and several medical journals devoted exclusively to the subject, doctors have started to move beyond this narrow-minded thinking. When you read a news article with the phrase "pain med use on the rise" it's not because we're becoming a nation of drug addicts, but rather that more and more doctors are getting comfortable prescribing appropriate pain drugs to help manage long-term chronic pain *not* caused by cancer.

In my view, using opioids for chronic non-cancer pain is probably one of the most significant medical breakthroughs of the past ten years. We've learning that the much-feared patient addiction rate (in some studies less than 1%) can be kept extremely low simply by keeping doses low.

I'm pleased to say that a majority of chronic-pain patients are quite responsible about medications, especially when their pain is finally brought under control. People in constant pain who are finally pain-free after months or years of misery simply don't want to endanger the relationship with their physician or with the medicines that help them live more normal lives. Are these patients addicts? Of course not. If they express anxiety about not being able to obtain their pain drugs (for example, if their doctor retired or they lost their health insurance), it's because they remember the pain and don't want to return to those days.

But bear in mind: more is not better in the world of pain management. For fibro patients, already hyper chemically-sensitive, my experience is that low doses go a long way toward effective pain control.

How the government's war on drugs changed doctors' prescribing

Unfortunately, the federal government's overenthusiastic war on drugs has frightened many physicians into simply not prescribing pain drugs to anyone, regardless the circumstances. Many pain prescriptions are classified as controlled substances, requiring all sorts of record-keeping on the part of physicians and pharmacists. I personally have no problem with this. There's so much paperwork running a medical office anyway that a few more minutes every day is no problem.

I can even appreciate the government-run online prescription tracking system for controlled medications — very Big Brother, but really it's better that a medical professional keep a watchful eye on her patient's prescription use.

However, because a few bad-apple physicians have been caught operating so-called pill mills (where pain meds are dispensed without adequate patient screening), the Drug Enforcement Administration (DEA) has established policies that can potentially criminalize any physician who writes pain prescriptions for his or her patients. When doctors read stories of new "pain patients" actually being undercover agents in disguise, capable of issuing arrest and search warrants, seizing assets, or threatening their livelihoods, even compassionate and reasonable physicians might simply say, "Pain management? I won't get involved."

Despite these significant roadblocks, the medical profession in general is heading toward a more enlightened use of pain medications. They're learning that these drugs are much safer than they were taught in school. For example, pill for pill, codeine is actually safer than ibuprofen because of ibuprofen's very real potential to harm the stomach and kidneys. The FDA is in the process of reformulating Vicodin (made up of hydrocodone with acetaminophen—i.e., Tylenol) to reduce the amount of the liver-toxic Tylenol in it, leaving the hydrocodone alone.

Rational doctors understand that no one needs to be in pain anymore. But despite the progress there is still one terrible, prevailing glitch in pain management. One elephant remains in the room.

When it comes to effective and lasting pain management, the sign on the doctor's door might as well read "Men Only"

I heard you gasp. Yes, it's true, and quite well documented in medical journals. Women are the losers when it comes to getting adequate pain relief.

There are two major reasons for this. First, the nearly worldwide societal attitude toward women in pain— whether from childbirth, menstrual cramps, arthritis, an autoimmune disorder, or any chronic illness. It's best described by the word "sexism." If you're a woman, expect to get the short end of the sympathy stick from your friends, family, and co-workers.

And from your doctor, expect that same short end when it comes to pain control. Consciously or unconsciously, the message to women in pain is: Live with it. The number of women in chronic pain who have internalized this message and said to me some variation of "I didn't want to bother anybody" is heartbreaking.

Young girls pick up on the minimizing of "girl pain" early in life. Sister's sports injury couldn't possibly be as painful as brother's, because, well, she didn't (shouldn't?) play as hard. Menstrual cramps can be so painful they cause some girls to faint, but when they seek help they hear a variation of "Take ibuprofen and get used to it." (Subtext: Honey, this is just a preview of what's ahead in your life. Just hope you don't get fibro.)

Along the way there's a curious irony. Women pay a price for being more articulate, more descriptive about their pain than men. Using more words to describe their pain and how it affects their lives is misinterpreted by a physician (usually male) as his patient being needy, whine-y, or just a plain old-fashioned hypochondriac. The doctor can better relate to a "real man" with "real pain" who is more likely to limit himself to "Hey, doc, my back really hurts, give me something for this, I gotta get to work" and his physician, admiring his patient's clipped stoicism, pleased with that masculine right-to-the-point, no-chatter attitude, rewards him with adequate pain control.

A woman with fibro, on the other hand, as she attempts to discuss with even a sympathetic physician the complexities of her pain and its relation to her life stresses, is often rewarded with a referral to a psychiatrist, her pain not addressed at all. At some time in the life of every fibro patient comes a moment when she leaves a physician's office with the sense that wherever the pain is coming from, and whatever the future holds, she's likely going to have to cope with it alone. She rarely learns exactly why her doctor can't, or even won't, help.

The second reason for the gender inequality in pain management returns us to the challenge all fibro patients face with their doctors: No positive tests. Men, when they suffer chronic pain, usually have a "something" that can be seen on an x-ray or MRI scan. Something like a chronic back injury or an unsuccessful orthopedic surgery, many times the consequence of a historical event like a fall from a ladder, playing rough sports in their youth, or a work-related injury.

With fibro, of course, there's nothing for the doctor to see in a test result, and therefore "nothing to treat." The doctor must take the patient at her word when she says she's in pain. And when it comes to prescribing pain drugs, most physicians are very reluctant to prescribe based on description alone, even after a fibro tender-point examination leaves their patient grimacing in pain. "Anyone can be a drama queen when I press tender points," a physician said to me recently after one of my fibro lectures to professionals. "How do I know she's not faking it just to get the meds?"

Keep in mind the numbers. There are 12 million people with fibro in the US, and 95% are female. Inadequate pain control by the medical profession should be as important a topic for women as abortion rights, unequal wages, child support, and abuse.

Why pain control is essential for most people with fibro

Laura's story clearly illustrates the necessity of adequate fibro pain coverage, her distress melting away with the Vicodin, her body able to stop holding itself rigidly against the pain. Did Vicodin cure her fibro? Of course not. Four hours after taking the Vicodin her pain would return. But remember, fibromyalgia is not a disease to "cure" but a chronic pain condition triggered by stress.

For Laura, unchecked pain contributed mightily to her stress. In fact, the original stress triggers that got her fibro going in the first place had long since receded. But now her stressors are the pain and an unsympathetic health care system (physicians, pharmacists, anti-drug chiropractors). Taking her Vicodin and feeling her pain melt away gives her hope, reduces stress, and sends the message to her body that the stress>pain>more stress>more pain cycle can be broken.

So let me re-phrase the answer to "Does Vicodin cure fibro?" No. Vicodin can't change your genetic susceptibility to the "pain amplification" issue of fibro, but adequate pain relief can go a long way toward lowering the volume on pain and bringing some joy back into life. Laura still needs to do the same fundamental work as you, moving through the weeks of the Nearly Natural Cure (page 103)—journaling, nightly hot soaks, guided meditation, stress reduction, starting gentle exercise, tracking symptoms, following the eating plan. But at least she can do these without her muscles being wracked with pain.

Still, it's important to remember that not everyone with

fibromyalgia needs pain drugs. For clarification on this, read How to Classify Your Fibro Severity (page 47) to determine which group you fall into.

I view prescribing opioids with the same seriousness as most physicians. The difference is that I will do it when needed. People with moderate fibro often need an opioid or opioid-like medication (tramadol) and those with severe fibro almost always do.

Given the changing, yet still-dim, views on pain meds held by most physicians, I can pretty much guarantee you'll never find anything like this section on opioids in any other fibro book. Nevertheless, some doctors are writing opioid prescriptions for fibromyalgia. Not long ago I was travelling with a drug company rep, on my way to give a fibromyalgia talk to a group of physicians. I asked him if the fibro diagnosis was being more widely acknowledged and how it was being treated in this particular area of the country. He pulled out his laptop "We're not supposed to show this," he began (showing me the "this") "but our company tracks what doctors in any area are prescribing for any particular condition. The pharmacies and insurance companies supply the data and apparently it costs a mint. Look," he pointed to a chart, "Vicodin and tramadol. The doctors *aren't telling anyone this. We get this data from the patients telling their pharmacists.*"

Opioids for fibro pain control

The numerous opioid medications are among the oldest drugs in the world and all work essentially the same way — by changing the way your brain processes signals of pain from anywhere in your body. Taking one these medications will reduce your perception of pain, increase your tolerance to pain, and decrease your reaction to pain.

Remember that because you have fibro, your brain overreacts to physical sensations ("pain amplification"). Your child's hug, your husband's affectionate knee squeeze, and countless other harmless events are felt by you as pain.

If the FDA-approved fibro medicines (see Medications for Fibro: How They Work and How They Can Help, page 187) are designed to ease pain then why do some fibro patients need pain drugs? For an unfortunately large number of people, the fibro drugs are simply intolerable due to side effects. We can't leave these people behind, and that's why opioids are sometimes necessary.

Another large group of people with fibro is able to tolerate one of the FDA-approved fibro drugs, but their pain is so severe that these meds are inadequate. Opioids are for them as well.

Side effects of opioids...and the risk of dependence

Taken at higher doses, the various opioids have largely the same side effects, including skin itching, nausea, dizziness, drowsiness, vomiting, constipation, physical dependence, and slowed breathing.

At the much smaller doses I prescribe, the sedation, dizziness, and nausea generally go away after a few days and in many people are avoided altogether. Constipation is the most stubborn of the bunch, and to avoid it many doctors prescribe a daily mild laxative like Senokot or Peri-Colace. I recommend All Bran cereal decorated with cut-up prunes.

Physical dependence, in which you crave the drug for the

drug's sake, virtually never occurs at low doses. What's interesting is that psychological dependence, which comes about from the fear of not having the med and having the pain return in full force, is very common.

Sadly, psychological dependence is mistaken for physical dependence by many doctors and when a concerned patient asks for OxyContin, she is often accused of what's commonly called "drug-seeking physical dependence" and humiliated by physicians, nurses, and pharmacists. If this happens to you, you need to find a new physician. For help, check these websites and be sure to give your new doctor the Physician's Guide to Fibromyalgia (page 299 + a printable PDF version at our website, wholehealthchicago.com):
— www.co-cure.org/Good-Doc.htm (fibromyalgia good doctor list)
— www.fmaware.org (National Fibromyalgia Association— click on "Healthcare Provider Directory")

Some people simply cannot tolerate opioids at any dose, experiencing unacceptable nausea and vomiting. Where your tolerance lies will be as individual as you. However, because with fibro you're more chemically sensitive than most people you'll react differently to the opioid family, and this actually can work to your advantage.

As you've probably guessed, because of your sensitivity to chemicals your likelihood of experiencing one of the side effects is increased, but this sensitivity works to your benefit as well. A small dose of any of these meds can go a long way toward helping reduce your pain.

Start low, go slow
Virtually all doctors who prescribe drugs for chronic pain follow the "start low, go slow" rule, increasing the dose

gradually until you report your pain is coming under control. This phrase "under control" is significant and should be interpreted as pain you find tolerable, pain you can live with. Some residual fibro pain will likely remain, but there are ways to control it *other than continuing to increase pain meds.*

That distinction is important. With fibro pain, "more" pain medication is definitely "not better." You can in fact become addicted to opioid drugs when they're steadily (and often thoughtlessly) increased to cover every last bit of pain. Don't anticipate total erasure of all pain. Down that path lies trouble.

With progressively higher doses, drug tolerance can also develop, the medication actually working less effectively to control your pain than it did at the beginning in a smaller dose. So by taking more of the drug you actually accomplish less, the treacherous path to overuse and addiction. Understand the line between correctly using pain medication and becoming addicted to it is easily crossed by asking your doctor for more and more pain drugs. Don't do it. I assure you that you don't want to become addicted to them.

Your goal is to break the stress>pain>more stress>more pain cycle that defines your fibro before you start reducing your pain drugs at the earliest opportunity.

Doctors like me who are willing to prescribe opioid pain medications for fibro usually have certain rules, and it's good for you to know them up front. Here they are:

- **Physicians prescribe a one-month supply at a time.** With lower potency pain pills (Vicodin, Butrans) refills may be permitted on the original prescription. Other drugs require a new paper prescription each month, in which case your doctor cannot phone refills to the pharmacy or fax a prescription. You will need a fresh prescription every month.

- **The physician's office must be in compliance with opioid regulations.** Your doctor's office will always know how many pills you have and you will not be allowed early refills without discussing the reason for this with your doctor.

- **You're not permitted to get pain medications from any other physician.** Most states have online systems to track this and virtually all physicians "fire" any patient who tries to break this rule (for obvious reasons).

- **You must never stop taking any opioid drug abruptly.** Doing so can trigger withdrawal symptoms (nausea as well as a surge of returning pain). If you want to stop taking a drug, ask your doctor for a schedule for tapering down your dose.

All opioid medications currently available are synthetic forms of codeine and morphine. Once absorbed by your body, the molecule travels through your bloodstream to specific "landing sites" in your brain called opioid receptors, at which point you feel less pain.

Which opioid medicines can work for fibro?
Opioids are commonly divided into three groups based on their length of action. Short-acting (lasting about 3 to 4 hours), long-acting (lasting 10 to 12 hours), and very long-acting (lasting 3 to 7 days).

Because people with fibro can experience pain 24/7, the longer-acting medicines can provide real relief from relentless discomfort without popping pills all day long.

Here's the low-dosing approach I use with my patients:

- I start by prescribing Tramadol ER (extended release).

- If it's not working, we switch to OxyContin 10 mg every 12 hours. This low dose rarely causes side effects, but may not be adequate for pain control either. The purpose of this approach is for you to be able to tolerate a larger dose if needed. If I prescribed OxyContin 20 mg every 12 hours immediately, you'd likely feel ill (with nausea and vomiting). 20 mg every 12 hours is the most common dose to control fibro pain, but it's certainly not needed if you have moderate fibro. If you have severe fibro (see How to Classify Your Fibro Severity, page 47) you may need to move to the 20-mg dose.

Tramadol (brand name Ultram) This is a synthetic form of codeine and widely used for fibro. In addition to acting on opioid receptor sites, tramadol raises levels of both norepinephrine and serotonin, similar to the FDA-approved fibro drugs Cymbalta and Savella. Given these three separate effects, tramadol sounds like the perfect medication for fibro pain control and many patients swear by it, especially the long-acting form, Tramadol ER (ER=Extended Release).

Tramadol ER is supposed to last 24 hours, but most patients report that it wears off by evening. Taking Tramadol ER 100 mg every 12 hours might work better than Tramadol ER 200 mg once a day. There is also a form of Tramadol combined with acetaminophen (i.e., Tylenol) called Ultracet, but I discourage my patients from using it because of acetaminophen's potentially toxic effect on the liver.

OxyContin (*oxycodone continual release*) is a time-release form of Percocet without the acetaminophen. It's highly unfortunate that this very excellent pain medication, requiring just one tablet every 12 hours (producing easy 24-hour pain control), has gained such a terrible reputation, including the criminalizing of doctors who prescribe it and their patients who need it.

OxyContin comes in tablets of 10, 15, 20, 30, 40, 60, 80, and 160 milligrams.

90% of my fibro patients get excellent relief by taking one 20-mg tablet every 12 hours, the same as taking a Percocet every four hours but without the returning surge of pain as it wears off. (To put this dose in perspective, according to news reports, Rush Limbaugh was taking up to *30 tablets a day* of whatever size OxyContin he was able to illegally purchase.)

After several months of pain control, many fibro patients are ready to try a lower dose, or want to get off it altogether. The fibro pain cycle has ended for them. Similar to OxyContin are Opana ER (time-release synthetic morphine) and Kadian (time-release morphine).

Vicodin (hydrocodone plus acetaminophen, very similar to Norco) is probably the most commonly prescribed synthetic opioid for common pain and is widely used for fibro. The main problem with Vicodin for fibro is that for many patients it lasts only about three hours and then rather abruptly stops providing pain relief. When that occurs, there is an all-too-human tendency to take more (and then, more) and one morning you realize you're taking quite a bit of Vicodin every day.

I limit my prescribing of Vicodin for our fibro patients to a maximum of three tablets a day. Many patients do nicely on this modest schedule and never require an increase. One or two tablets of Vicodin per day are allowable while also using OxyContin to cover a phenomenon called breakthrough pain, which can occur when using one of the longer-acting opioids described here.

The FDA is in the process of getting Vicodin manufacturers to reduce the amount of acetaminophen in its pills, which, considering its liver toxicity, is a good idea. Slightly stronger than Vicodin is another synthetic opioid, Percocet (oxycodone plus acetaminophen).

Duragesic (fentanyl) is a synthetic opioid absorbed though your skin after applying it as an adhesive patch that you change every three days. Duragesic comes in several sizes, from 12.5 mcg/hr (micrograms of medicine released per hour) through 100 mcg/hr. Most fibro patients get good relief with the 25 mcg/hr size.

Butrans (buprenorphine) is another synthetic opioid absorbed through the skin via an adhesive patch. With Butrans, you change the patch weekly, so your doctor's monthly prescription will be for four patches. Unlike other opioids, physicians are allowed to write refills for Butrans. The patches come in 5-mg, 10-mg, and 20-mg sizes. Most of our fibro patients have done nicely using the 5-mg or 10-mg size.

I can't say if your personal physician will be willing to write an opioid prescription for fibro pain control. Your best bet may be to start with your family physician since he or she has likely known you the longest. Share with your doctor the physician's guide at the end of this book (also available as a printable PDF at our website, wholehealthchicago.com), which includes my recommended dosing and rationale behind it. If your family doctor isn't any help, try a pain specialist or a rheumatologist.

12

ALTERNATIVE MEDICINE FOR FIBROMYALGIA

Despite your physical misery, fibro's not directly dangerous to your health in the way that a condition like high blood pressure is. And it's because of this that you're afforded the special opportunity of going slowly and trying a variety of different therapies, some considered "alternative" by doctors.

Understand that conventional physicians fall across a philosophical spectrum in their views of using alternative medicine, ranging from the sensible ("It won't hurt to try") to the unreasonable ("They're all quackery"). Happily, over the past 20 years, as more and more physicians learned about the diverse fields encompassed by alternative medicine, many have come to see that a blend of both conventional and alternative is an ideal approach for people suffering chronic symptoms, especially when prescription drugs are getting them nowhere.

For your fibro, in addition to the lifestyle changes and supplements suggested in the Nearly Natural Cure (page 103), you're free to work with virtually any alternative therapy, and this is also true even if you're taking prescription drugs. One essential fact about the vast majority of alternative therapies: they're extremely safe.

The choice is always yours. Whether you want to work with conventional medicine alone, alternative medicine only, or blend the two, the most important idea is for you to do *something* for your fibro. Some of you may have already started regular exercise, others a weekly massage. Maybe you're regularly sweltering in the heat of Bikram yoga (page 130) or devoting your free time learning everything you can about fibro. Good work—you're all improving your situation.

Choosing to do anything won't damage you or worsen your fibro and, in fact the only decision that would actually make matters worse is doing nothing at all. Sitting around watching TV, limiting activity to refilling your Pringles bowl, and feeling sorry for yourself because you're tired and you hurt is a prescription for everything getting worse. So take the first step now and review this section to see what resonates with you as an approach that might help.

Alternative practitioners

The spectrum of alternative practitioners I've collaborated with over the last couple decades includes massage therapists and other bodyworkers, physical therapists, chiropractors, acupuncturists, and various energy healers including Reiki practitioners. Although each of these fields has its own explanation for *why* fibro develops in a person, their success rate for helping people with fibro is also quite high, not least because alternative practitioners are a compassionate group known to spend more time with patients than most hurried conventional physicians who may not "believe" in fibro at the outset.

It's possible that working with any of the following alternative medicine areas could improve your fibro to the degree you feel nothing else is needed. For a good example of this, read about Brigadier General Becky Halstead on this page.

Patient Stories: How Chiropractic Helped A Brigadier General's Fibro

Severe fibro symptoms forced Brigadier General Becky Halstead into early retirement from the US Army and out of the Middle East.

"Agonizing pain, debilitating fatigue, joint stiffness and sleep deprivation—you name it and I felt it," she told a reporter. "There I was in Iraq, responsible for over 20,000 military men and women, and I privately struggled to physically keep myself going."

These days, however, she feels quite well, attributing her pain-free health and conquest of fibro to saying "no," better nutrition, and chiropractic, so much so that she's become a spokesperson for the profession.

From what you've read elsewhere in this book, you can probably guess how her fibro got started. Brigadier General notwithstanding, she was a low-serotonin woman who after 27 years of service, many in battle zones, finally surpassed her stress-buffering system. Her muscles locked into a protective suit of armor and she developed fibro.

It's not surprising that the fibro rate among US troops overseas, male and female alike, is quite high.

Returning stateside, the general's stress level plummeted. She made some key choices, her chiropractor loosened her taut muscles, and life once again was restored to her.

The right alternative modality for you and your fibro depends largely on personal preference. If you were raised in a home where your parents regularly went to a chiropractor, then you'll likely feel comfortable working with one. Conversely, if you're needle-phobic, acupuncture is probably not a good choice, no matter how enthusiastic your friend might be about her new acupuncturist. If you unabashedly feel connections with spirituality and healing energies, then by all means consider Reiki or Healing Touch. On the other hand, if your take on fibro focuses more on body mechanics, skip the Reiki and head for chiropractic, physical therapy, or bodywork therapies like myofascial release.

The primary disadvantage of alternative medicine therapies is that their beneficial effects can be short-lived. Notice I didn't say "are short-lived." Some of my patients feel great after a massage, chiropractic adjustment, acupuncture, or Reiki, but after a few days their muscle pain starts to return. Your experience may differ.

From my own integrative perspective, I'd urge you to use the Nearly Natural Cure (page 103), with or without prescription medications, along with an alternative therapy you feel comfortable with. Six to eight weeks of intensive weekly therapy seems to be the magic number. After this, many patients experience such considerable improvement that some therapies can be reduced to monthly treatments or eliminated altogether.

Physical Therapy

You might think it odd to begin with physical therapy (PT), now so common on the healthcare landscape that very few people, physicians included, regard physical therapists as alternative in any way. But strictly speaking, they're classed as alternative health care providers.

Most physical therapists are taught something about fibro during their training — probably quite a bit more than most

MDs, actually. However, because their treatments are limited to PT modalities, most know little about other treatments, either conventional (like medications) or alternative (nutritional supplements, Chinese medicine, etc.)

Usually you arrive in a PT office with your doctor's prescription, which states your diagnosis and lists some specific therapies. If no therapies are prescribed, your doctor may prescribe a more open-ended "Please evaluate and treat."

Physical therapists do treat large numbers of fibro patients and many of them are quite good at it. They use a variety of approaches including massage, myofascial release, heat, ultrasound, and therapeutic exercises.

Advantages There are about 150,000 physical therapists in the US, so you won't have to go far to locate one. Also, if you have health insurance your doctor can write a prescription for PT and either your therapist will bill your insurer directly or you'll be reimbursed for some of your expenses when you submit a claim.

Disadvantages Like everything else in health care, the quality of PT can vary widely. Some PT offices are oriented toward treating injuries or strokes, and the therapists are more focused on this kind of rehabilitation. In such settings, therapists are able to treat up to four patients at a time using weights, exercise equipment, and so forth. A fibro patient requires longer visits and more individual attention, so you might do well to seek out a therapist who works in her own office and has a special interest in fibro. A second disadvantage of PT is price, so if you don't have health insurance, economically you may be better off seeing a massage therapist or myofascial release therapist and paying less out of your own pocket.

Chiropractic

Because chiropractors specialize in diseases and disorders of the musculoskeletal system with special emphasis on the spine, they are likely treating far more fibro patients than conventional physicians. Moreover, surveys have shown a very high patient satisfaction rate with chiropractic and quite a few patients, like Brigadier General Halstead, rely heavily on their chiropractors to get over fibro flares.

In the view of some chiropractors, called "straights," fibro occurs solely because of a misalignment of the spine. Using spinal adjustments along with a variety of therapeutic modalities, they believe that if these adjustments can "hold," your fibro can start clearing up by itself. More holistically oriented chiropractors, called "mixers," believe that stress has tightened your muscles and subsequently misaligned your spine, and that both issues need to be addressed. You probably gather that I am more in tune with this second group.

Nevertheless, having a chiropractor on your fibro team is a good idea (we certainly have them for our fibro patients at WholeHealth Chicago). I'd also bet that your chiropractor would more readily read the accompanying Physician's Guide (page 299 + available as a printable PDF at our website, wholehealthchicago.com) than your primary care physician, be amenable to ordering the neurotransmitter and adrenal profiles from NeuroScience, and be especially pleased to learn NeuroScience has a Professional Education module that teaches any interested physician how to incorporate nutritional supplements into treatment.

A chiropractor would also be more familiar than your regular doctor with the supplements in the Nearly Natural Cure (page 103).

Like physical therapists, chiropractors use a wide variety of therapeutic modalities. In addition to an assortment of hands-on treatments, your chiropractor may use ultrasound, infrared, electrostimulation, and acupuncture. Many chiropractic offices have massage and myofascial release therapists as well.

Advantages With more than 50,000 chiropractors practicing in the US, every small town and every big city neighborhood has at least one. Most health insurance policies now cover chiropractic and the practitioners themselves are quite good at getting reimbursements for many of their treatments, including massage and myofascial release.

Disadvantages Like their MD counterparts, many chiropractors still "don't believe in fibro" and spend years (and a lot of their patient's money) trying to get the spine in alignment, the adjustment to "hold." A good number of my fibro patients have told me they simply gave up after a couple of years of weekly chiropractic treatments.

The problem is that most chiropractors are unaware of the serotonin/stress susceptibility aspect of fibro and also how exactly the FDA-approved fibro drugs (Savella, Cymbalta, and Lyrica) actually work.

Because the central philosophy of chiropractic defines it as a drugless therapy, some chiropractors, though certainly not a majority, throw the baby out with the bath water and discourage all prescription meds, even for fibro patients. For years, their professional association gave out bumper stickers reading "Say no to ALL Drugs" with an Rx encircled in red and crossed out with the familiar slash. This is where you, as a proactive person with fibro, can make a key choice: If chiropractic seems to be helping but you feel you need a little more help, follow the Nearly Natural Cure and/or ask your physician to prescribe one of the fibro drugs discussed on page 197.

Eastern Medicine

What I've described so far looks at fibro from the perspective of Western medicine, are all based on human physiology—your physical self—and what can go wrong with it.

However, traditional health care practitioners from the East—China, Japan, southeast Asia, and the Indian subcontinent—have a different perspective on health and illness. As such, their treatment of what we in the West call fibro is radically different from ours. It's not a question of which is best, since both systems of care can be effective. Rather, it's more an issue of where your personal preferences lie, based on the culture you grew up in as well as your life outlook.

Generally, throughout the East both good health and illness are integrally tied to an invisible energy force, variously called qi (pronounced "chee") in China, ki in Japan, and prana in India. This subtle energy courses through the universe and through all animate and inanimate objects. If you're a healthy person, this force—your qi—flows smoothly through your body along channels called meridians. Conversely, ill health comes about by imbalances, blockages, and stagnations of your qi.

When you visit a practitioner of traditional Chinese medicine, she'll take a complete medical history and examine your tongue and pulse to determine the status of your qi.

Chinese medicine practitioners attempt to restore to balance to your qi, both by inserting acupuncture needles along specific pathways of qi flow called meridians and with individually formulated herbal blends.

Reiki, Healing Touch, and Ayurvedic practitioners do comparable energy shifting with their hands. A Reiki therapist or Ayurvedic practitioner will hold her hands an inch or two above your body and literally *feel* the shift in energy, sensing imbalances in your energy centers, called chakras.

Whether energies run along meridians or via chakras, the principles remain the same. When your energies are balanced and flowing smoothly, good health will follow.

Advantages Traditional Chinese medicine, Reiki, Healing Touch, and Ayurvedic medicine are all extremely safe and can be used alone or in combination with Western medicine. Although much is made about potential interactions between Chinese herbs and prescription drugs, they virtually never occur.

Disadvantages Finding qualified practitioners may be challenging. If you're interested in working with Eastern medicine, find a practitioner fully certified in both traditional Chinese medicine and Chinese herbs. Some physicians and chiropractors have taken courses in acupuncture, but it doesn't come close to the education of a certified practitioner. Practitioners of Reiki, Healing Touch, and Therapeutic Touch can now be found in almost every community.

Another disadvantage is cost, as virtually none of these therapies is covered by health insurance. If your employer has set up a health savings account system, you can receive some reimbursement through it.

Bodywork therapies, especially
myofascial release

There are dozens of bodywork therapies and once, trying to list them all, I reached about 50 and simply stopped counting (just google "bodywork therapies" and you'll see what I mean"). Although no form of bodywork is harmful in any way, as a person with fibro you'll discover that some are more effective than others, and that within each particular therapy much of the benefit lies in the skill of the therapist.

Although you'll certainly enjoy some temporary relief of symptoms from getting a simple massage at a day spa, if you want to make real progress and spend your health care dollar wisely, I recommend finding a therapist who's been professionally trained to treat fibro.

By far the most helpful of the bodywork therapies for fibro is myofascial release therapy, part of your assignment in Week 1 of the Nearly Natural Cure (page 103).

A myofascial release therapist is usually a physical therapist or massage therapist who has taken extra coursework. Don't feel at all reluctant to ask about her training, her experience with fibro, and what techniques she'll use during a treatment session. Most myofascial release therapists I've spoken with are quite aware that releasing tightened fascia can bring up deeply buried emotional issues in their client. Even though they're not trained psychologists, they'll work diligently to help you feel safe and secure during your session.

As you'll recall, fascia is the fibrous covering of muscles. With fibro, as muscles tighten throughout your body the coating of fascia tightens as well. Simply massaging the tightened muscles helps loosen those painful knots you feel and will certainly give you temporary relief, but for long-term benefit the tightly wrapped fascia itself needs to be stretched — unwound, really — to allow muscles to move normally and blood to circulate freely within them.

In the system first described by Wilhelm Reich, emphasis is placed on muscle "memory," literally trapped emotional trauma that needs to be released for healing to begin. Let me say here that this concept is so essential to your fibro recovery that I wrote an entire chapter on it (Memories in Your Muscles, page 57).

Your muscles once learned to tighten up in response to a traumatic event. Now, although that event is long forgotten (or repressed), your fascia is tightly locked and your muscles continue to respond to stresses of any kind by contracting further. Myofascial release therapy breaks this cycle.

There are two forms of myofascial release therapy, direct and indirect. Therapists are trained in both forms and use one or the other depending on the situation. Direct myofascial release is also known as deep tissue work, during which you lie on a massage table and the therapist, using tools like knuckles, elbows, rollers, or rounded wooden or plastic knobs, presses firmly into your tight fascia and muscle knots until they're stretched, lengthened, and loosened.

Note: if you have severe fibro you won't want to start with direct therapy (too painful). Instead, you'll want the therapist to use indirect techniques.

Indirect myofascial therapy, which was first described in the 19th century by osteopathy founder Andrew Taylor Still, MD DO, is more a gentle stretching of tight muscles (and subsequently the fascia) across a path of least resistance. The therapist begins by actually feeling areas of inappropriately tight fascia with her hands, which for most fibro patients starts in the neck, shoulders, and upper back.

Having perceived an area of taut fascia, she'll stretch it herself until she encounters a barrier or restriction to the movement. At that point, she'll pull a little further at the muscle beneath the fascia, "holding the stretch" herself, for 3 to 5 minutes. The fascia will actually resist this stretch initially, and as it does she'll be able to feel it generating a slight pulsating heat. As the restriction releases, the therapist will feel the movement give way and the fascia soften. Ultimately, repetitions of sustained stretch and pressure will loosen the fascia over your entire body and dramatically help your fibro.

Advantages You shouldn't have any difficulty finding a myofascial release therapist, and if your doctor is willing to write you a prescription for myofascial release therapy your insurance (assuming you have some) can offset some of your expenses. If your doctor won't write a prescription for it, see Week 1 of the Nearly Natural Cure (page 103) for help finding a new doctor.

Disadvantages Some patients with severe fibromyalgia find that any sort of bodywork therapy, including myofascial release, is simply too painful. If this applies to you, I suggest starting with a combination of medication and Healing Touch or Reiki. During these energy therapy sessions, your practitioner's hands are held either very slightly above your body or, at most, rest painlessly on your body. In either case, the sessions are completely painless.

13

YOU'VE GOT A FRIEND: WOMEN SPEAK OUT ABOUT THEIR FIBRO

During one week in May, 2010, more than 500 women with fibro participated in an online survey, a joint effort of healthywomen.org (a leading online health website for women) and Harris Interactive Service Bureau (a survey company). The research on the project and its results was coordinated by Edelman StrategyOne, a public relations firm, and funded by Forest Laboratories, a pharmaceutical company that had recently released Savella, one of the three FDA-approved medications for fibro.

I'd been sent the results of this survey in November, 2010, and was asked if I would discuss them with the media. Those of you who know and read my weekly health tips understand I'm no booster for the pharmaceutical industry. From "creating" diseases in order to sell drugs to other dirty tricks, my issues with Big Pharma are well known.

But this was different. This was about fibro, whose very existence is doubted by highly educated physicians. This was about women with fibro all over the country (and world, via internet) hearing a doctor (me) discussing the survey results and saying yes, absolutely fibro is real and makes your hurt. I'd be acting as a sort of bullhorn for the voices of 500 women with fibro who had taken the survey. Along the way, maybe a lot of physicians would hear those voices as well.

Helping the patient teach her doctor

Also, this gig would be different than many set up by Big Pharma and here's why: the policy of Forest Labs is to shun all direct-to-consumer TV, magazine, or newspaper advertising. Instead, their marketing division decided the best way to teach doctors about fibro would be the campaign to let women with fibro know that (a) they weren't alone, and (b) medications were available to help them.

Armed with information, fibro sufferers would then theoretically elbow their way into their doctors' offices and ask about the chances their symptoms were caused by fibro. With any luck, the doctor would respond, "Why, yes, I've been hearing a lot about it lately" and consider prescribing one of the fibro drugs.

Even if the doctor ultimately prescribed a competing drug, Forest Labs figured, at least fibro was now on this doc's diagnostic radar screen. On the other hand, if the doc snorted, "There's no such thing as fibromyalgia," the patient could always find another doctor to ask for treatment.

This seemed eminently sensible to me. Neither I nor Forest Labs wanted the public release of this survey to be a commercial. If a reporter were to ask questions about specific fibro medications, I would name all three of the FDA-approved fibro drugs. It was also fine with Forest Labs that I talk about the alternative therapies you'll be using in the Nearly Natural Cure (page 103) that forms the centerpiece of this book.

Any physician who's had experience with what fibro

patients endure would not be surprised at the results, and you with your fibromyalgia won't be either. However, everyone at healthywomen.org, Edelman, and Forest Labs seemed shocked by the extent to which fibro affected women's lives and the struggles they endure to get help from the medical profession. The responses from magazine reporters were a pretty uniform, "Wow! These are scary numbers!"

After I completed nearly 60 TV, radio, and magazine interviews, internet activity for the word "fibromyalgia" dramatically increased and apparently has remained that way. I'm hopeful the strategy of helping the patient teach her doctor is working.

Let's review the key findings of the WE FEEL survey

WE FEEL stands for Women Expressing Fibromyalgia's Effects on their Everyday Lives (who thinks of these things?). Remember, these are the answers to a series of fibro-related questions from 500 women who have already been diagnosed with fibro. Keep in mind that this is a tiny sample out of approximately 12 million American women (and 200 million women around the world) with fibro, 90% of whom remain undiagnosed.

In the US, this means that 12 million women spend their days in 24/7 chronic pain. That's roughly eight times the population of my beloved sweet home Chicago. Pretty staggering numbers, though nothing new to you if you're struggling with fibro.

Read through the summary statements here (in bold), derived from the information given by those 500 women.

The quotations that follow each statement are from fibro patients themselves. I can already see you nodding in agreement, echoing these sentiments and feelings. At least you know you're not alone.

Fibromyalgia is a significant burden on patients, with 85% considering it a major burden on their lives and 86% reporting symptoms in the moderate-to-severe category.

- "The pain has taken over my life. I dream of waking up in the morning, jumping out of bed in no pain at all, and going out for a run. Instead I lie there, feeling my muscles throb."

- "I try to put on my happy pain-free mask when I'm with my family, but they can tell."

- "I guess I must move like a 90-year-old, but I'm only 30."

- "I sat on the sofa crying and crying and my husband just sat there helplessly. I finally screamed, 'I am SO TIRED of hurting.'"

Nearly half (47%) of those surveyed reported their work or career had been negatively affected by fibromyalgia. Two-thirds (67%) said they could no longer keep up with household chores because of their fibro.

- "At first my employer started making concessions because she'd read about fibro, but then there were just too many absences. I was falling behind, and knew I had to quit."

- "When I applied for short-term disability, I was told there was no such thing as fibromyalgia."

- "I look around the house and see the mess. I clean a little and then just sit there. I'm so tired that the thought of shopping for groceries and making dinner is overwhelming."

- "My husband is really supportive, but I know he must be hiding his disappointment in me. He works all day, comes home to help with dinner, and in the evening, I'm in bed by 8."

Because of their fibromyalgia, two women in five (42%) spend less quality time with friends, one in three (29%) spend less quality time with family, nearly one-third (31%) said fibromyalgia affected their ability to experience intimacy.

- "There's nothing quite as awful as having to gently push your child away just because she wants to give you a hug. But with fibro, hugs hurt."

- "I never can play with my children. They know that 'mommy's sick.' Their friends all know that I'm the Sick Mommy."

- "We haven't done anything in the evenings for years. Too tired."

- "Enjoy sex? You've got to be kidding. Sometimes if I find the right position it isn't too bad."

Ask Dr E: How do I explain fibro to my children?

With children, keep it simple and not frightening. Fibro is not being sick, like when kids have the flu, so there should be no "Mom's got a sickness" language, which could cause your children unnecessary worry.

Every child understands the phrase "Mommy's tired, honey" and also knows to ease off and let Mommy rest for while.

Unfortunately for some moms with fibro, it really hurts to hug or be hugged by anyone. Again, common sense says not to be overly dramatic when your child wants a hug. Say something like, "Mommy's arms are hurting today, so let's see how gently you can hug me."

Kids learn quickly that dad gets the hard squeezes and mom the gentle ones.

May I emphasize here how important it is for you to take care of yourself? Many women put family before their own health, and in your case this could produce a real reversal in any progress you're making. Stay on my plan, making healthful eating and gentle exercise a priority along with the nightly relaxing bath and other steps outlined in the Nearly Natural Cure (page 103). Your partner should also read about fibro to understand your symptoms and physical limitations.

Every fibro patient needs to recognize that her symptoms, though not an actual disease, are a message from her body asking for a change. The first step for many is learning the correct pronunciation of the word "No," as in "No, I just can't do it/attend/volunteer/take on the extra work."

Fibromyalgia asks that you resign from being super-mom and just be mom.

Most patients suffer for years. Seven in ten (71%) did not seek help until their symptoms became intolerable. For more than half (54%), once they did seek help, the diagnosis took a year or more. One respondent in four (23%) said it took multiple physicians five years to make a diagnosis. This confirms a previous study in which patients reported needing to see five physicians before they were diagnosed with fibromyalgia. Half the respondents believe the delay in their diagnosis was due to their physician's lack of knowledge about fibromyalgia, the other half believed it was their own lack of knowledge.

- "I was told I was developing early arthritis and to take aspirin and live with it."

- "My doctor said I was just being lazy."

- "The rheumatologist said I was just depressed and to see a psychiatrist. The psychiatrist said there was nothing wrong with me but gave me an antidepressant anyway. Nothing happened so I stopped taking it."

- "The only time my pain actually stopped was when I had root canal work and my dentist gave me some Vicodin. I mentioned this to my doctor and he said if I took more, I might become a drug addict."

- "One doctor did give me a pain pill and it really helped. Once when I went to fill the prescription, the pharmacist wanted to know if I had cancer. I burst into tears. Very embarrassing. Does he think I like taking pain pills every day?"

- "My chiropractor said there was no such thing as fibromyalgia and that my spine was misaligned. He signed me up for a year's worth of adjustments. I'd get one or two days of relief from an adjustment, but then back to square one. Finally I gave up on that, too."

- "One rheumatologist said I had some kind of autoimmune disease and put me on some medications that had terrible side effects. When I looked at my tests, they were all negative. I wonder what he was thinking."

- "When what I now know was fibromyalgia was affecting my pelvic muscles, my doctor wanted to perform a hysterectomy. I decided against that."

- "Back when I first had what I later learned was fibromyalgia, nobody knew about it. I had all this pain in my neck and shoulders. An orthopedic surgeon decided it was due to my bulging discs, so I had a lot of surgery on my spine. Of course, three months later, same pain as before the surgery."

A medical system unresponsive to 12 million women

These are brutal and disturbing statistics. It's astonishing that the medical profession can so preoccupy itself, fine tuning the management of conditions that have virtually no symptoms (high blood pressure, diabetes, high cholesterol, obesity) and yet sit in stony silence, unresponsive to the needs of 12 million women experiencing constant widespread muscle pain.

Back to the survey results...

Fibromyalgia patients face skepticism about their condition. 64% believe their condition is not taken seriously by anyone. When seeking a healthcare provider, 79% of women surveyed specifically seek a doctor who will take them seriously.

- "A neurologist actually said to me that fibromyalgia was an imaginary condition for Caucasian women to avoid housework."

- "I once saw a play where one of the characters had fibromyalgia. When the husband in the play said 'My wife is having problems with her fibromyalgia," everybody laughed. The playwright had actually meant this to be a funny line."

- "I was told fibromyalgia was an imaginary condition

until Blue Cross denied me health coverage. I said 'But I was told it wasn't real!' and they said it was on their list of 'uncover able conditions,' which at least proved to me it *was* an actual condition."

- "The nurse from the disability insurance company called to check on me and then muttered, 'Fibromyalgia? Bet you're just sitting around eating bon-bons. You're lucky to have fibromyalgia." I started crying on the phone and she hung up."

Below, two comments from my own experience that shocked me:

- From a gynecologist: "I'd yank a woman's uterus out before I'd start her on pain meds for fibromyalgia."

- From a 4th year medical student rotating through our integrative health clinic, WholeHealth Chicago: "I've never heard of fibromyalgia except on TV commercials."

Early diagnosis is important...and a huge relief

91% of the women in this survey reported feeling relieved when they could finally connect a condition to their symptoms. I'm hopeful if you haven't yet been diagnosed but sense from this book that you do have fibro you'll find similar comfort in just knowing what it is you've got.

If this describes you, turn to the Nearly Natural Cure for help finding a physician who can properly diagnose you so you can begin treatment as soon as possible. This is essential, as the survey also showed that women who were diagnosed and started treatment earlier (within a year of their symptoms starting) were less likely to experience significant challenges to their careers, families, and relationships.

This echoes the experience with my own patients. I know when fibro is diagnosed sooner it's far easier for my patient and I to treat it than it is for those with longstanding fibro. By the time a woman's had fibro for a decade or longer, her muscles and the fascia covering the muscles are so locked up that more modest fibro treatment simply isn't as effective. More potent approaches, including medications, need to be introduced.

As a way of underscoring the strength of the link between your mind and body, let me close with an e-mail from a patient. I clearly recall her palpable relief when I told her she had fibro...and that it was reversible. I think it says worlds about the importance of just *knowing*:

"Thank you so much for explaining fibromyalgia to me and giving me a plan of action. I know the plan could not have taken effect this soon, but you've got to believe I am actually feeling a little better already."

14

FIBRO'S LARGER MESSAGE: WOMEN UNDER SIEGE (OR WHAT WOMEN ENDURE LIVING ON A GUY'S PLANET)

I sometimes wonder if women have become almost numb to the violence directed against them, the day-to-day stress they face. If you're a server in a restaurant, an irate customer will yell at you but remain silent before the six-foot-tall male maitre d'. You'll be passed over by your university tenure committee even though you've been voted "most popular professor" and have published nationally read academic research. The guy sitting next to you at your job, whose work is marginal at best, gets promoted to an office with a door, not you, whose work has been rated consistently outstanding.

Last year I saw a pretty terrible movie based on what I've heard is a remarkable book, *The Girl with the Dragon Tattoo*. Watching the film, you could guess the villain in the first 30 minutes. But also after 30 minutes, I would have expected women in the audience to walk out en masse. That's because in less than an hour, Lisbeth Salander (the one with the tattoo), had endured sadistic beating, forced fellatio, and anal rape. By the end of the film, she'd uncovered a serial killer and the audience was treated to extremely graphic photos of women decapitated, smothered, and cut in half, sliced like prime rib.

Yet when I asked the women in our office what they thought of the film, most said, "Yeah, pretty good. The book was much better." I asked if any had been offended by the sadistic depictions of women. They blinked at me with a look that said, "Hmm, must have missed that."

Now it's worth mentioning that the book's author, the late Stieg Larsson, deliberately wrote Lisbeth Salander as a powerful and independent female protagonist to express his own anger about violence against women. Indeed, everyone who crosses Ms Salander comes to a bad end.

But in the day before writing this, I'd seen the now-famous photo of the beautiful Afghan girl whose nose and ears were cut off by her husband, read about a woman stoned by the Taliban for adultery, and noted that Newt Gingrich, having abandoned his first wife when she was diagnosed with cancer, had walked out on his second wife for a younger third.

I learned that the economic recession was responsible for overcrowded women's shelters (women fleeing to escape their abusive husbands) and read a seemingly tongue-in-cheek article on how the Chicago's apparent serial wife-killer Drew Peterson is dealing with life in jail. Also in that day's paper, more about the infamous Craigslist killer, who lured women to their deaths by advertising online.

Over the next few weeks (and sadly with no great effort), I gathered articles on worldwide violence against women: Bride burning in India and Pakistan, hundreds of "honor killings" in the Muslim world, clitorectomy in Africa, and sex trafficking in Bangkok, midtown Manhattan, and Des Moines. There were stories on the millions of rape victims who are part of the "spoils of war" and the astonishing work inequality in developing countries (everywhere I travel, men seem to loll around drinking mint tea or coffee while women do everything else).

Gender-based violence looks like a womb-to-tomb affair. Consider the fate of vast numbers of female infants in China, the murder rate of young women who fail to give birth to sons in Pakistan.

Violence directed toward women seems endless and utterly senseless, occurring in every segment of society regardless of culture, class, or ethnicity. War and economic recession simply crank up the volume.

And while pretty much your entire low-serotonin gender is more sensitive to all this stress than the male half of the planet, roughly 10 to 15% of women are especially serotonin-deficient, acting as the canaries in the coal mine for the rest. Remember the vulnerable canary? Coal miners, when testing a mine for poison gas, would lower a caged canary down the shaft. These birds are exceedingly sensitive to the effects of gas, and when the cage was pulled up, if the canary was dead the miners stayed away from that toxic spot.

The larger message of fibro is this

You and your entire sisterhood have been under siege and you've been so since you were born. How you as a unique individual respond to this siege depends primarily on two factors: the strength of your stress-buffering serotonin system and the severity of the stress itself.

Variability in this regard is as diverse as the population of women and the broad range of stressful factors affecting them. You may get debilitating migraines from a change in barometric pressure or a fibro flare-up when your partner complains you're not holding up your end of the bargain. You might feel a knot in your stomach when you hear a child cry or clench your jaw when someone makes a joke about a minority.

Wherever stress-buffering is low and stress is high and lasting, look for fibro and the fibro spectrum disorders, muscles painfully tightening against an emotionally toxic environment. For women without fibro, try to be there for your sisters. Because for those who have fibro, the world is even more hostile.

And with all that in mind, fibro truly becomes a metaphor for a woman's predicament on planet Earth. No condition in the history of medicine demands so much of its sufferers, who must be proactive, demanding, feisty, and angry...just to get treatment.

Throughout this book I've referred to fibro and its spectrum of related conditions as low-serotonin disorders. Many times you've heard me say that women are the ones who get fibro because their stress-buffering serotonin is so much lower than that of men. Stress exceeds the buffer, your fight-or-flight response triggers muscles to painfully contract, your stress-coping adrenal glands become exhausted, and there you have fibro in a nutshell.

Among the central treatments in my nearly Natural Cure, I hammer away about lowering stress levels and boosting serotonin, emphasizing the necessity of enhancing your stress buffer to quiet your body's endless fibro pain/stress cycle.

But let's shift the prism a couple degrees and look at all this from a slightly different perspective. What does the fact that

95% of people with fibro are women have to tell us about the position of women on our planet? Virtually all cases of fibro begin after several months of unfettered, intense stress in a woman's life. In addition, epidemiologic studies repeatedly confirm that every fifth fibro patient was sexually or otherwise physically abused as a child or young woman.

A hostile world toward women

From wage inequality at one end of the spectrum to stoning for being a "disobedient" wife, women must always be on the alert for trouble from men. Whether it's a slap from an abusive boyfriend, a mugging in Central Park, a date rape in an otherwise Norman Rockwellian suburb, or the anxiety a single woman feels wondering who's really going to show up for her internet date, women live forever on the alert, with a largely internalized yet persistent sense of fear.

Just like all employees carry the relentless worry that they might get fired, women are ever-poised for trouble from earth's other gender, one poisoned with too much testosterone and granted more muscle mass than is good for it.

The indifference of the male-dominated medical profession — and the financial priorities of the similarly male-dominated pharmaceutical, health, and disability insurance industries — have contributed mightily to make the fibro situation worse. Add to this the isolation felt by most women with fibro due to friends and family members who, consciously or not, notice she "doesn't look sick" and puzzle that her "tests are all negative," which must mean nothing really serious is going on.

What proportion of fibro stress comes from inequality — from relationships between men and women, the shifting roles of women and men in contemporary society, the stubborn and serious inequities in women's compensation for equal work?

How much fibro is exacerbated by a less-than-empathetic medical system?

Little wonder the main feature of fibro is the constant tightening of the muscles that wrap around your body, like a mummy enclosure ever-tightening in an effort to protect you from this hostile world. As we discussed in Memories in Your Muscles, this is the unconscious creation of a suit of armor using muscles, first described in the 1920s by psychiatrist Wilhelm Reich, who termed it character armoring.

All women are under constant siege.
From men.

Here am I, a male physician, my gender controlling the government, medical profession, pharmaceutical industry, health and disability insurance industries, and probably your workplace too.

Men's so-called normal serotonin levels protect us from the stress that we ourselves have largely foisted on the world, with women suffering the consequences, assaulted by the horrors that my gender creates but can tolerate.

I occasionally wonder what would happen if somebody added serotonin-boosting Prozac (or Savella or Cymbalta) to our water supply. The 12 million US women with fibro, and untold millions suffering low-serotonin depression, anxiety, OCD, PTSD, TMJ, tension and migraine headaches, irritable bowel syndrome, and chronic fatigue syndrome, would get their serotonin bumped up and might be more adequately armed to cope with the stressors of a world run by men.

Of course, women's pathetically inadequate serotonin levels are genetic and you just keep passing on this susceptibility to your daughters. Your misery goes on for generations. Good thing we doctors (still mostly men) and the pharmaceutical industry (absolutely mostly men) have come up with some chemicals for you to take. Good thing you've got health insurance (more men still), because these drugs are expensive. If you don't, you'll simply suffer, because even more men will vote against universal health care and your disability insurance (just guess who runs that shady industry) will deny your benefits because fibro "isn't real" in the first place.

Am I hearing stirrings of anger? Or is it the sound of you massaging your painful shoulders, that aching neck?

Wait. I hear a voice from the back of the room.

"Just a minute, Edelberg," rising and rubbing out painful fibro knots in the back of her neck, a smart feminist snarls back at me, "My serotonin level is just fine. You with your super-serotonin, you're both a bully and an emotional zombie. War is a guy thing, and so is wife beating. You may love your dog, but you'll blow a deer to kingdom come on opening day of hunting season. Intuitive skills? You've got the intuition of a cement block."

As her muscles loosen, she takes a breath. "Listen, doc, not having such a spectacular stress-buffering system keeps me in touch with the world, protects me from being like you. At least I'm intuitive, sensitive to colors, textures, sensations, and I can negotiate disagreements instead of making a fist or getting my stealth bombers lined up. I bet your poor wife rolls her eyes to the ceiling as yet again she explains the patently obvious to you. I don't terrorize weak people, like women, children, and the oppressed. And I can cry, and most of you men can't or won't. And I can love deeply in ways that you can only read about."

And now, finger jabbing the air, aimed at me. "You have the balls, sorry, the temerity, the nerve, to brush me off with an antidepressant. Something to bump up my stress buffer so I can be an insensitive and violent clod like you? Please. Why don't you take something, invent a pill to lower your own serotonin? Make you more sensitive to the world. Maybe it'll make a nicer guy out of you. Maybe you'll think twice before you call in the army to kill women and children."

"Well, yes," I stammer. "All true." Leaving this imaginary auditorium, I mull over her words. And undeniably I feel a wholesale embarrassment for my entire gender.

It gets worse for women

Then one morning I open the Chicago Sun-Times to see photos of two young women who had been beaten senseless by a male attacker wielding an aluminum baseball bat. The paper specified aluminum because it's so much harder than a wooden bat, itself no Twinkie when smashed into your skull. He'd wanted their iPod. The two women had been admitted to an intensive care unit and their conditions were "guarded."

I imagined comments from police and tsk-tsking from others, "Well, they shouldn't have been out walking in the middle of the night. And carrying an iPod. What were they thinking?" If you are inept at finding a criminal, it's quick and easy to blame the victim.

"It is," I think to myself, "very, very rough being a woman."

In fact, after some thought I couldn't come up with a single aspect of my own life that wasn't easier simply because I'm a guy. I've never been underpaid because I'm female, never sexually harassed. I've not had my career stymied by an old boy's club. I can go into a bar for a martini and nobody ever hits on me. I don't look over my shoulder walking home from a movie at night. Rapists do not stalk middle-aged Jewish guy doctors.

"In fact," I think, "if I had to endure what women put up with, day in and day out, I'd go bonkers." And at the word bonkers, I consider the larger idea of "mental illness" as it relates to women and their low serotonin stress-buffering systems.

Is one entire gender making the other emotionally and physically ill? Is that's what's going on, and fibro simply the most visible manifestation of this worldwide epidemic?

I think that's a large part of it.

As the feminist pointed out to me, the problem is not really that a woman's serotonin is too low, but rather that men have too much. We're overly buffered against stress. We've been rendered numb, insensitive, and clueless. "Numb," by the way, is a word I frequently hear when a woman's dose of a serotonin-booster like Prozac or Lexapro is too high. She's become one of us, one of the pod people from "Invasion of the Body Snatchers." She'll say, "I've become a zombie. I don't laugh or cry." My response to her: "Welcome to Guyville (and, by the way, let's lower your dose)."

It gets worse. When men drive you up the wall, and you hate the very sight of us because of insensitive cluelessness, women lack equal upper-body strength to lob a well-deserved punch in our collective snouts. If you were just a bit stronger, you could grab our neckties and scream, "Stop your guy nonsense! You idiots are destroying the world. You invade countries, you kill people, you beat wives, steal pension funds, and bang women over their heads for an iPod. Rather than invent new medications to raise our serotonin, find something to lower yours! (And while you're at it, do something about all that testosterone, too.)"

The health consequences of stress

Endlessly throttled by all this male-created stress, women become emotionally and physically ill (as any sane person would). You visit your physician, are told your test results are normal and that you're depressed, and are handed one of the many pharmaceuticals that will raise your serotonin, so you can be more resilient, "tougher," and able to endure the hostile, violent world we force you to inhabit. Since you can't lick us, take some Prozac and join us.

Along the way, your utterly appropriate emotional responses to this insane world earn you the various labels of mental illness. You'll be diagnosed as "depressed," "anxious," "phobic," "paranoid" — all these from a (male-written) psychiatric diagnostic guide. Post traumatic stress disorder? Where do these guys think your trauma came from?

But ponder this: It used to be worse, much worse. Up until about 1950 or so, before mind-controlling chemicals, if you were a women and miserable with your thankless life in a sweatshop or as unpaid slave labor at home, your (male) doctor simply certified you as insane and you joined tens of thousands of your sisters in residential mega-psychiatric hospitals for the rest of your life.

A couple of years ago, I went to see a new play called "The

Walls." Lisa Dillman and the company members of Rivendell Theatre Group created a very dramatic and troubling work about women as victims of involuntary psychiatric hospital admission. Back then they called it involuntary "commitment" as in "being committed to a mental institution."

What was extremely painful about "The Walls" is its historical accuracy. Dillman followed the lives of three women, one from the late 19th century, one from the 1930s, and one young woman who easily could have been sharing a seat with you on the bus this morning.

Few people are aware of the magnitude of gender-biased involuntary psychiatric confinement that existed until about the 1960s. State psychiatric hospitals, like Manteno in downstate Illinois, contained thousands of patients in huge dormitory facilities. The hellishness of these places was the subject of the 1948 film The Snake Pit, and as a result of the film's widespread audience reaction many of the hospitals were either closed or underwent significant rehabilitation.

Psychotropic medications had not been discovered, so patients with diagnoses like depression (then called melancholia), anxiety (hysteria), and schizophrenia (dementia praecox) did not receive Lexapro, Xanax, or Risperdal to normalize their serotonin or calm them enough to allow them to endure "normal" lives in a world they simply could not tolerate.

Instead they were swept up and confined, often for decades, abandoned by families who wanted to deny any insanity in the family. It's hard to grasp how many of these women must also have suffered from relentless and utterly untreated fibro and chronic fatigue as well.

Women medicated

It doesn't take a lot of imagination to wonder why the majority of patients receiving "help" for mental illness have always been women. During the 1960s psychiatrist Thomas Szasz, MD, took the medical profession to task in his book, *The Myth of Mental Illness*, for its very loose standards in diagnosing mental illness. How much depression, anxiety, even schizophrenia was, in fact, the only way a woman could cope with a deeply troubling and hostile world?

How much mental illness is simply a failure to conform to the male standards of behavior? Emotionally troubled men and women exist in a world where conformity is rewarded. Over the years, non-conformity was treated first by institutionalization, then by lobotomies, and recently by lots of medication.

Although antidepressants can be miracle drugs in the right situation, doctors vastly overprescribe them to women for symptoms that are simply part of life (a relationship break-up, loss of a beloved pet). And the health insurance industry strongly encourages automatic renewals of antidepressants to avoid paying for psychotherapy. A year's worth of Prozac costs around $60, about half the price of a single session of psychotherapy.

You have to wonder how many medications are prescribed because a woman is not conforming to the male ideal of "woman." How much of a woman's allegedly errant behavior occurred because she perceives the insanity of her life? How many prescriptions written because her male physician wanted her to be more like his own idealized image of himself (strong, tough, unemotional).

Although I write a great deal in this book about drugs for

fibromyalgia, both FDA-approved (Lyrica, Savella, Cymbalta) and off-label, I fully realize that I'm writing about chemicals that alter brain chemistry so that half the Earth's inhabitants can endure what the other half has done to them and to the planet itself. I am also fully cognizant that the muscular armor of fibromyalgia is essentially a complex coping mechanism to protect a woman from all this madness.

With one published study showing that 70% of antidepressants for depression and anxiety were inappropriately prescribed, it does seem a large portion of "mental illness" among women just might be a male-created myth, a deliberate conspiracy now profitably exploited by the male-dominated medical, insurance, and pharmaceutical industries. Numbing women with drugs makes a whole lot more financial sense than institutionalizing them…or making the world a better place for both sexes.

Had the Neanderthal not been a hunter—but rather a farmer who never needed a perversely high stress buffer—and everyone's serotonin was low like women's (i.e., normal), today's men might be more intuitive, sensitive, and gentle. Perhaps they'd even be ashamed to use baseball bats when they went out at night hunting for an iPod.

15

A BRIEF HISTORY OF FIBROMYALGIA

The two most famous historical figures who had what we'd likely diagnose today as fibromyalgia were inarguably also the victims of chronic stress. As you'll read throughout this book, stress pulls the trigger on fibro, starting it up and keeping it simmering.

First, from the Bible poor Job, pawn of the superpowers, his life a perfect storm of stress as his faith is relentlessly tested, bemoans "I, too, have been assigned months of futility, long and weary nights of misery. When I go to bed, I think, 'When will it be morning?' But the night drags on and I toss until dawn...Depression haunts my days. My weary nights are filled with pain as though something were relentlessly gnawing at my bones." (Job 7:3-4 and 30:16-17)

Fast-forward to the 19th century and we get the first inklings about what would ultimately be named fibromyalgia in 1976. The first full fibro description was written by William Balfour, MD, at the University of Edinburgh in 1816, what he called "muscular rheumatism." Eight years later he added the locations of the famous fibromyalgia diagnostic tender points.

Meanwhile, caught in the front lines of the Crimean War in 1854, her own life constantly in danger, nurse Florence

Nightingale developed all the symptoms of fibromyalgia and chronic fatigue. Her condition was so severe that on returning to England she spent the last 50 years of her life virtually bedbound. Hers was "muscular rheumatism with neurasthenia." Different words, same condition.

By reading the Victorians—and not only medical articles, but also the popular press, novels, poems, and plays—we start to see how fibromyalgia and chronic fatigue began to dramatically interfere with people's (mainly women's) lives. In 1813, the London *Examiner* accused as its cause the "present luxurious age remarkable for its nervousness," and by the 1860s psychiatrists felt that modern civilization made for nervousness, that anxiety was everywhere. Throughout Europe and the US doctors believed the stresses of modern life were causing an epidemic of "nervous exhaustion." As a result, furniture makers created chaise lounges and fainting couches.

The "stress of modern civilization"
In a popular medical book of the time, *A Practical Treatise on Nervous Exhaustion (Neurasthenia): Its Symptoms, Nature, Sequences, Treatment (1881)*, George Miller Beard, MD, lists symptoms including insomnia, flushing, drowsiness, bad dreams, cerebral irritation, pain, pressure and heaviness in the head, and sweating hands and a smorgasbord of phobias, including open places, closed places, society, contamination, and "fear of everything," along with utter and complete exhaustion (neurasthenia). The pain component was variously termed "muscular rheumatism," "hysterical paroxysm," and "psychogenic rheumatism."

Beard felt the condition arose from modern civilization, and both Victorian women and their physicians agreed that the hustle and bustle of everyday life was too much for women, and their susceptibilities to stress, to endure. The idea that the perils of modern life were simply unendurable caught the imagination on both sides of the Atlantic and there is no shortage of 19th century novels and plays in which women of all ages "collapse" from an exhaustion that physicians, more than 100 years later, would attribute to adrenal burn-out.

By the end of the 19th century, psychiatrist Sigmund Freud would begin to write about the suffering of neurasthenia. Initially, he joined the crowd who believed the exhaustion was a historical phenomenon, the "stress" of contemporary times, but later Feud would add that many physical symptoms were caused by the excessive sexual repression of Victorian middle-class women. Today, despite the great credit virtually all psychologists give Freud for his theories on the subconscious, everyone largely concurs that repressed sexuality is passé as a touchstone for all our anxieties. Nevertheless, Freud did agree that susceptibility to stress, especially for women, produced significant symptoms, both emotional and physical.

Around the same time that Freud was writing about the effects of stress, English physician Sir William Gower noted that neurasthenia was often accompanied by the presence of muscular rheumatism and its tender points, believing the muscles were actually inflamed. He coined the term fibrositis in 1904. Medical terminology adds "-itis" to any organ believed inflamed, as in tonsillitis, appendicitis, and dermatitis.

And 70 years later...

For nearly 70 years, fibrositis remained in place, but by 1976, never having found any evidence of actual inflammation in the muscles, the name was changed to fibromyalgia, the Greek word for muscle pain. When "-algia" is added to a body part, it simply means pain (next time you have a headache, tell everyone you have cephalgia).

Still, because of its utter absence of positive test results, it wasn't until 1981 that the first controlled study describing symptoms and tender points was published. Then, in 1987 the AMA recognized fibromyalgia as a real condition (despite the absence of positive test results) and in 1990 Frederick Wolfe, MD, was lead author on a position paper of the American College of Rheumatology that defined fibromyalgia on the basis of symptoms plus tender points.

From the moment the paper was published, a majority of American physicians were (and remain) very skeptical about whether or not fibromyalgia deserved to be its own clinical entity. Having normal blood tests, x rays, CT and MRI scans, and even muscle biopsies, most doctors, including myself, despite all the symptoms women experience from fibromyalgia, are reluctant to call fibromyalgia a "disease," in the way say, rheumatoid arthritis, lupus, osteoarthritis, and so forth, are diseases.

Even Dr Wolfe, more than 20 years later, no longer calls fibro a disease, believing, "the tendency to respond with distress to physical and emotional stressors is part of the human condition."

I agree, but with this added caveat: Yes, stress may be part of the human condition, but women face far more day-to-day stress and are less well equipped biochemically to defend themselves from it. And that's why 95% of all fibro patients are women.

You'll read much more about all this in other chapters.

16

PREVENTING
FIBROMYALGIA

Given that fibro affects up to 7% of all women in the US (about 12 million people, more than have diabetes), there's been remarkably little written about prevention. If you've arrived here before reading the rest of the book, I recommend you do that now to gain a clearer idea of how fibro starts, gets a foothold, and won't let go.

Medicine's near-wholesale failure to understand this once-puzzling condition is the likely reason prevention hasn't been adequately addressed. To the detriment of the millions of women living with fibro, the vast majority of physicians at one time simply doubted there was any condition to begin with. Their attitude was: Why bother thinking about preventing something that isn't real anyway? Just send these pesky patients to a psychiatrist.

The handful of doctors who "believed" fibro existed knew it was somehow a cousin to depression and stress, but didn't understand exactly how these branches on the family tree intertwined. But now that we know a lot more about fibro these connections have been made, and it's true that just as diabetes can be prevented, so can fibro.

Happily, an increasing number of physicians are saying to themselves, "Ah! Now I can grasp how this fibro puzzle fits together." As a proactive fibro patient, you need to understand this too.

What we know about fibro and the fibromyalgia spectrum

We definitely know that women are at greatest risk for fibro, and we also know why—because of a genetic predisposition that leaves them more vulnerable to stress. The most common fibro triggers (stress and physical injury, the latter another form of stress) are also recognized, and everyone is disturbed about the statistic that 25% of women with fibro experienced pretty brutal childhoods.

Although chronic muscle pain, exhaustion, poor sleep, and brain fog are the hallmarks of fibro and enough for any human being to endure, many woman later diagnosed with fibro first experienced a group of seemingly unrelated symptoms, now called the fibromyalgia spectrum. These symptoms can appear years before the widespread muscle pain of fibro begins, or they can occur right alongside fibromyalgia.

With a history of any of the following fibro spectrum symptoms, you are vulnerable to developing fibro. But there are lifestyle changes that will protect you, and we'll discuss these further below.

Symptoms of the fibromyalgia spectrum

Understand that each of these fibro spectrum symptoms is caused by low levels of the neurotransmitter serotonin, which buffers stress. Many times in this book you'll hear me say that women are the ones who get fibro because their serotonin levels are so much lower than those of men.

When stress exceeds your buffer, your fight-or-flight response triggers muscles to painfully contract, stress-coping adrenal glands become exhausted, and there you have fibro in a nutshell. These conditions are all related to stress and low serotonin (as is fibro itself).

- A sense of profound exhaustion.
- Sleep that's not very refreshing.
- Brain fog.
- Depression.
- PMS.
- Anxiety.
- Obsessive thinking/compulsive behavior.
- Tension headaches (squeezing tight-band headaches).
- Migraine headaches (throbbing, often with nausea).
- Irritable bowel syndrome.
- Eating disorders.
- Post traumatic stress disorder.
- Jaw clenching (temporomandibular joint disorder— TMJ).
- Symptoms worse in winter (seasonal affective disorder— SAD) and during your premenstrual week.
- Carbohydrate craving with weight gain.
- Chronic pelvic pain.
- Lack of sex drive.
- Painful intercourse.

Take this quick quiz to gauge your fibro risk

To prevent fibro you must first determine if you, as a unique individual, are at risk for developing it at some point in your life. Take this quiz to find out.

Are you female?
Y – N

Have you experienced any of the following or has any female relative (to whom you're biologically related) been affected by any of these:

Depression or generalized anxiety disorder
Y – N

Chronic carrying of stress in neck and upper back
Y – N

Chronic tension and/or migraine headaches
Y – N

Irritable bowel syndrome
Y – N

Chronic pelvic pain with no obvious cause ever found
Y – N

Jaw clenching (TMJ)
Y – N

History of injury to the neck or spine from which you feel you've never completely recovered (the whiplash injury that "never seemed to go away")
Y – N

Emotional, physical, or sexual abuse during childhood
Y – N

Seasonal affective disorder
Y – N

Taken SSRI antidepressants (Prozac, Celexa, Lexapro, Zoloft, Luvox, Effexor) and obtained good results. (These medicines raise serotonin. If your symptoms improved on any of these, we can assume you are a low-serotonin, stress-susceptible person.)
Y – N

Multiple chemical sensitivities (certain scents make you feel sick) and susceptible to the side effects of drugs
Y – N

Do you regard yourself as being more sensitive to the world or to stress in general than other people you know?
Y – N

KEY

Low risk If you answered "no" to everything except being female, you're at extremely low risk for ever developing fibro.

Moderate risk Answering yes to up to 5 questions places you at moderate risk for fibro.

High risk Answering yes to 6 or more questions places you in a high-risk category, especially if you answered yes to the final question. Fibro patients are exquisitely sensitive human beings and they discover, often in childhood, that the world surrounding them is a rough place to exist.

Facts about fibro

From what you've read in this book about fibro, you know that:

- Fibro is not a disease but rather the result of an unchecked "fight-or-flight" stress response.

- Fibro involves the brain chemical (neurotransmitter) serotonin, which acts as a stress buffer.

- Serotonin levels are lower in women than men. Based on an inherited, genetic predisposition, some women have extremely low serotonin levels.

- These women, when confronted with prolonged stress, can develop one or more of the low serotonin stress susceptibility disorders in the fibro spectrum. Fibromyalgia is one of these.

- Unchecked stress depletes your stress-response glands — your thyroid and adrenal glands — and this depletion is the main cause of the fatigue that accompanies fibro.

Five steps to preventing fibro

Keeping these fibro facts in mind, here's my prescription for fibro prevention.

Manage stress Always be aware that you are more susceptible to stress than others. At each of the many decision points in your life, base your answer on one criterion only: will it cause me more stress or less stress? More stress is a deal-breaker, whether this decision relates to job, relationship, or any responsibility. Did you know low-serotonin women possess superior intuitive and observational skills? Take advantage of these. If your intuition is screaming, "Don't do it!" you'd better not be nodding your head yes.

Next steps: Read through the Nearly Natural Cure (page 103) for help with stress reduction. You'll find a constellation of ideas—from the nightly hot soak in your bathtub and eliminating foods that stress your body to the guided meditation that will take you far far away from whatever's stressing you.

Avoid overdoing As a corollary, learn the correct pronunciation of the word "no" as in "No, I'm really sorry I can't/don't have time for that." Overscheduling your life puts you on the fast track for a tsunami of stress, adrenal gland depletion (and subsequent exhaustion), sleep deprivation, and poor nutrition.

Next steps: Read Structuring a Life Without Fibro (page 131) and take each step to heart.

Boost your low serotonin Every single day of your life, be aware of your low serotonin status and take these positive steps to shore it up:

- Regular daily exercise is the very best way to boost serotonin, even if it just means going for a walk.

- Get into the sun, avoiding sunglasses for at least part of the time. Your brain makes serotonin when sunlight enters your eyes.

- Consider yoga classes. They boost serotonin, lower stress, and stretch tight muscles.

- Take every day of vacation you're entitled to.

- Unless you really dislike animals, consider getting a pet (reports show that pets can lift serotonin).

Next steps: Read and follow the Fibro-Friendly Eating Plan (page 145). It's a way of maximizing foods that raise serotonin while reducing the serotonin-busting action of sugar and other fast carbs. This will lower your risk for fibro.

Explore unresolved life issues If you have significant biographical issues that you haven't explored, including coming from a stressful childhood or living through a stressful adulthood, consider talk therapy. Festering wounds affect a very real percentage of women with fibro and symptoms of the fibro spectrum. Resolving them keeps you healthy.

Next steps: Read Memories in Your Muscles (page 57) for a guided tour of your memory palace and how your muscles remember everything that's happened to you.

Pay attention to your early warning system Use messages from your body, especially coming from the muscles in your neck and upper back, as an early warning system that something in your life is out of balance, causing stress. When you feel these muscles tighten, start examining what's happening in your life. Then, move forward with getting this stress under control. Fibromyalgia-wise, ignoring these warnings is like taking your phone off the hook when someone is calling to tell you your house is burning down.

Next steps: Read about Eastern medicine and bodywork therapies in Alternative Medicine for Fibromyalgia (page 245). Getting some help for early signals from your muscles limits your risks for fibro and fibro spectrum disorders.

Fibro Quicksand: Ignoring symptoms

Feeling chronically tired and achy? You need to be checked for fibromyalgia. If your own doctor doesn't know much about fibro or dismisses it altogether, see Week 1 in the Nearly Natural Cure (page 103) for help finding a new physician.

In a survey of people with fibro, 79% said a top issue was locating a doctor who would take their condition seriously.

Once your diagnosis has been established, consider the range of therapies outlined in this book—from supplements or prescription medications to physical therapy, healthful eating, yoga, and alternative therapies like acupuncture. All of them can help.

As you begin to understand fibro and its spectrum of symptoms, you'll become more successful in managing it. And because symptoms are generally triggered by stress, when a flare-up occurs, instead of feeling hopeless and helpless you can review your life for stress sources and renew your efforts to resolve them. Then, treat yourself to some pleasant treatments (regular hot soaks, massage, guided imagery, yoga), work with your doctor to adjust any medications you're taking, and move forward.

Ignoring symptoms will only keep you stuck where you are.

If, despite your best preventive efforts, you're feeling an increase in muscle pain and it's becoming more widespread, turn to How to Classify Your Fibro Severity (Chapter 5), focusing on the section on mild fibro. Then, take action with the suggestions outlines there.

Otherwise, do spend the remainder of your incarnation in prevention mode.

17

PHYSICIAN'S GUIDE TO FIBROMYALGIA

This short guide accompanies my patient-directed book *Healing Fibromyalgia*, which is based on my experience treating more than 1,600 fibro patients.

Because of the nature of this condition, and the frequent necessity of prescription drugs, I wasn't quite sure how to get the reader's primary care physician involved. Virtually all fibro patients need professional expertise at hand.

And then I thought: I'll write a short guide and offer it free. The book buyer can print it out and hand it to her doctor (you'll also find a printable PDF version at our website, wholehealthchicago.com).

And now, she and I have our collective fingers crossed that you'll read it.

In the very next section you'll encounter some startling facts about fibro, including these two: epidemiologists estimate 10 to 14 million people currently fulfill the accepted diagnostic criteria for fibro...and that about 80-90% of that group are undiagnosed.

This huge group of undiagnosed fibro patients are struggling mightily with their lives—family, relationships, careers, and activities of daily living all compromised by fibro.

For that reason and this one, I urge you to read this guide: a typical fibro patient suffers needlessly for five years and is seen by four physicians before someone says to her, "This looks like fibro."

You could be that doctor.

A fibro diagnosis is neither rare (more women have fibro than have diabetes) nor particularly difficult to make. I sketch out the protocols for you below. What sets fibro apart from the rest of what we all learned in medical school is that it is not a disease with abnormal tests and tissue pathology, but instead the normal physiologic fight-or-flight response gone utterly and completely awry.

This absence of positive tests has done a major disservice to fibro patients. They're endlessly told "we can't find anything wrong with you" and dismissed as chronic complainers.

Your patient bought the book because someone, perhaps you, told her she might have fibro. Maybe she pieced together symptoms that had been a mystery and diagnosed fibro herself (many women do). Perhaps the diagnosis was suggested by her chiropractor, massage therapist, or a friend. Possibly her sister was diagnosed with fibro and she realized she had the same symptoms herself...or she took an online quiz and her eyes widened when she read her score: You likely have fibromyalgia.

Twenty years ago, I decided to open a medical center that combined conventional and alternative therapies. As the internist, I was the "straight man" to a bevy of very interesting and compassionate "other" healers like chiropractors, acupuncturists, massage therapists, and herbalists.

Desperate for help, having been literally turned away from

conventional medical offices ("I think you should see a good psychiatrist"), women began arriving with longstanding fibro and chronic fatigue symptoms. These two conditions, essentially two sides of the same coin, have been our commonest diagnoses by far.

The protocols presented here are based on our 1,600 fibro patients and divided into mild, moderate, and severe categories. If you have any questions, I'm happy to hear from you.

David Edelberg, MD
WholeHealth Chicago
davidedelberg@hotmail.com

Part 1: What is Fibromyalgia?

Fibro is a chronic muscular pain syndrome. Based on what we all learned about *disease* in medical school, fibro is not a disease. The muscles in a fibro patient are completely normal. No enzyme elevation, no autoimmune antibodies, no abnormal nerve conduction. When biopsied, fibro muscles look like what they are: muscle.

The primary symptoms of fibro are chronic (over three months) widespread muscle pain, a sense of profound fatigue (previously known as chronic fatigue syndrome), and unrefreshing (non-restorative) sleep. For a condition as potentially disabling as fibro, it is astonishing that so many years elapsed between its original description in 1816, the criteria for diagnosis from the American College of Rheumatology in 1990, and the release of the first FDA-approved but decidedly problematic drugs (because of side effects) Lyrica ™, Savella ™, and Cymbalta™ in 2008 and 2009.

Even now, when I travel the country and give talks on fibro to physician groups, I am frequently met with skepticism about the very existence of this condition. Audience members who tell me they "never see any fibro patients" are discomfited to be told that statistically 7% of their female patients probably have fibro. What is going on here?

Let me review some interesting facts about fibro in terms of actual numbers:

- Epidemiologists estimate that 10 to 14 million people currently fulfill the accepted diagnostic criteria of fibro.

- Because there are no positive tests to diagnose fibro and a physician must rely on his or her clinical acumen, approximately 80-90% of these 10 to 14 million are undiagnosed, often for years.

- The condition occurs mainly in women (96%), approximately 7% of the female population of the US.

- More women have fibro than have diabetes.

- Fibro occurs world-wide, estimated to affect 200 million women on the planet.

- The disbelief in fibro's very existence among physicians comes from the flaw in medical education that in order to be real, a condition must have verifiable pathology, positive tests, or visible tissue pathology. Fibro has none of these.

The online survey called WE FEEL (Women Expressing Fibromyalgia's Effects on their Everyday Lives), conducted by Harris Interactive among 508 women diagnosed with fibro, revealed the following data:

- 85% of women with fibro consider it a significant burden in their lives.

- 64% felt their symptoms were not taken seriously by their health care provider.

- A typical fibro patient sees four separate physicians before she learns her diagnosis.

- Not infrequently, once a woman learns she has fibro she is told "we don't know much about this condition, there's not a lot to do for it."

- As her years with undiagnosed fibro continue, her symptoms progressively worsen. Most women wait for their symptoms to reach an intolerable level before seeking the right help and finally getting their diagnosis. This usually averages five years, but can take even longer.

- If treatment is delayed and symptoms are allowed to worsen, fibro becomes progressively more difficult to treat successfully. The three FDA-approved drugs demonstrate just a 45% success rate in relief of symptoms, and this 45% occurs in patients who have not suffered years and years of fibro.

- Fibro symptoms can begin at any age. Children as young as eight have been reported with fibro.

- Fibro severely impacts a woman's family life, her relationships, her career, and all activities of daily living.

The reason for the delay in making a fibro diagnosis is our own professional discomfort with this condition. One survey among physicians revealed that roughly 60 to 70% of physicians didn't feel confident when making a diagnosis of fibro. Fibro breaks the rules of how we were all taught to diagnose any condition. We were told that when a patient presents with symptoms, we begin by performing a physical examination and then, based on our working clinical diagnosis and our knowledge of pathophysiology, we order tests, including blood tests, imaging studies, and biopsies.

Positive test results confirm our clinical suspicions and we can begin appropriate treatment. *Negative test results* either steer us down an alternative diagnostic path or allow us to tell our patient the single most common sentence heard by fibro patients: We can't find anything wrong with you. All your tests are normal.

Sadly and often based on some serendipitously borderline positive lab test result, fibro patients are incorrectly misdiagnosed with an unrelated condition. It is not unusual to encounter fibro patients who have undergone needless surgery or received unnecessary medication. For example:

- A large rheumatology department near my office routinely starts fibro patients with weakly positive ANA levels on a lupus protocol.

- Patients are not uncommonly started on anti-inflammatory medications for alleged rheumatoid arthritis based on a borderline elevated sed rate (and negative rheumatoid factor).

- Chronic pelvic pain (a common fibro symptom) is treated as interstitial cystitis or even, if a small fibroid is noted on ultrasound, the patient is advised to have (and often undergoes) an utterly useless hysterectomy.

- Because of fibro tender points on the anterior chest wall, fibro patients have undergone coronary angiograms. One patient with fibro, panic attacks, and tachycardia underwent an ablation procedure.

- Patients undergo unnecessary (and always unsuccessful)

cervical and/or lumbar disc surgery with spinal fusion. Several years ago, one prominent group of neurosurgeons "discovered" that both fibro and chronic fatigue was caused the Chiari malformation (small foramen magnum pressing on the brain stem). Their barbaric procedure uselessly opened dozens of foramina. Naturally, no one improved.

Most commonly, fibro patients are simply written off as depressed. Of course, depression is a normal emotional response for anyone with untreated chronic pain and fatigue who has been told "nothing is wrong." Since SSRIs do have marginal benefits for fibro, the patient thinks "maybe I was just depressed after all" until her fibro starts getting worse. Psychiatrists regularly see patients with fibro referred to them by both primary care physicians and rheumatologists. They virtually never believe depression alone is responsible for all the symptoms experienced by the patient.

Fibromyalgia defined

If you ever hear someone say "We don't know the cause of fibro," don't accept that answer. We now know exactly what is happening with fibro, why some women are victims and others not. We know the physiology and we now have a good understanding of a variety of treatments and why and how these treatments work.

Fibro is a syndrome affecting primarily women who have a heightened sensitivity to painful stimuli (abnormal pain processing) and feel more pain to any noxious stimulus (pain amplification). A physician can observe these phenomena clinically by performing tender point examination (see below) or simply inflating a blood pressure cuff to 180 mm/Hg on a fibro patient. She will complain of significant pain and appear distressed (tearfulness, diaphoresis), while the same procedure done on a person without fibro causes no appreciable response. If, at a later date, the doctor were to ask "How long did your tender points hurt after the examination?" he or she shouldn't be surprised to hear the patient was uncomfortable for several hours.

A person's susceptibility to fibro is genetic and involves both diminished levels of the neurotransmitter serotonin and an increased release of pain transmitters (glutamate, substance P) per noxious stimuli.

Serotonin and its role in fibro

The neurotransmitter serotonin, present in both the central nervous system and the GI tract, acts as our "factory-installed" stress-buffering system. Likely as an effect of evolution, the male level of serotonin as stress buffer is three to four times that of a female. This means a woman is more susceptible to stress, both physically and emotionally.

Were we to measure serotonin levels in both men and women, we would see a pair of bell-shaped curves, some women in the "low-male" range, some men in "high-female."

It is the very low-serotonin women at the far left of the bell-shaped curve who are most vulnerable to stress. These women go through life like walking open wounds with the whole world as salt shaker. It is from this population we find the women most susceptible to developing fibro.

Low-serotonin stress susceptibility disorders
• Female predominance

- Familial disposition, multigenerational
- Usually triggered by stressful events in a woman's biography
- Can begin in childhood
- Worsen during winter (reduced sunlight reduces serotonin production)
- Worsen whenever blood levels of estrogen are diminishing (premenstrual days, postpartum, perimenopause)

Psychological manifestations of low-serotonin stress susceptibility disorders

- Depression
- Generalized anxiety disorder and/or panic attacks
- Obsessive thinking
- Compulsive behavior patterns
- Social anxiety disorder
- Post-traumatic stress disorder (especially abuse during childhood)
- Phobias

As every clinician has observed, after 4 to 6 weeks of treatment with any serotonin- enhancing medication, most patients report varying degrees of improvement. This is their stress buffer on the rise. It is accepted good medical practice that taking steps to lower stress through psychological counseling will enhance the effectiveness of antidepressant medication: Anxiety, depression — raise stress buffer (SSRI) + reduce stress (counseling) — clinical improvement

Women often unconsciously self-treat their low-serotonin symptoms with:

— Exercise (regular exercise raises serotonin)
— Sunlight (sun exposure raises serotonin)
— Carbohydrates (raise serotonin)

Physical manifestations of low-serotonin stress susceptibility disorders

A variety of physical symptoms often accompany the patient's psychological symptoms. Not infrequently, physical symptoms may be the only manifestation of "stress" exceeding the stress buffering system. These symptoms may be interpreted by both patient and physician as disease, but despite symptom severity tests are normal and no disease is found (unless a separate disease is found).

Physical symptoms are all part of the physiologic stress response, the fight-or-flight in a constant "on" state.

- Muscle tightness in neck and upper back ("I carry my stress in my neck and shoulders").
- Tension and migraine headaches.
- Jaw clenching, jaw grinding, and TMJ.
- Fibromyalgia itself ("My muscles are tight everywhere, like a suit of armor"). **See below for diagnostic criteria of fibromyalgia.**
- Irritable bowel syndrome (bloating, frequent indigestion, constipation, diarrhea, abdominal cramping).
- Chronic pelvic pain and dyspareunia.
- Premenstrual dysphoric disorder.

When to suspect fibromyalgia

Keep in mind that fibromyalgia is Greek for "muscle pain."

- Widespread symmetrical muscle pain present for longer than 3 months.

- Presence of anatomically defined "tender points" (see next section). A positive tender point means that significant pain is induced by 4.4 kg of fingertip pressure. Tender points *must have a left-right symmetry,* and *must be above and below the waistline.* The patient must demonstrate pain in 11 of the 18 defined tender points to fulfill the diagnostic requirements for fibro. (Note: the tender-point criteria remains useful despite being eliminated recently by the American College of Rheumatology as being too vague and subjective to establish a fibro diagnosis.)
- Muscle stiffness.
- Unrefreshing (non-restorative) sleep.
- Chronic tiredness (chronic fatigue syndrome).
- Decreased overall sense of well-being.
- Cognitive dysfunction ("fibro fog").
- Depression.
- Tenderness of musculoskeletal structures and skin.
- Persistence of pain after noxious stimuli ceases.
- Allodynia (pain from normally non-noxious stimuli).
- Family history of low-serotonin stress susceptibility issues.
- History of physical or sexual abuse as a child (applies to 25 to 30% of all fibro patients).
- No evidence of joint inflammation or positive lab test results.

Testing for tender points

Use the accompanying diagram to locate tender points. Place your index finger on a hard surface and press until blood is drained from your nail bed. This is approximately 4.4 kg of pressure.

Press each of the tender points with 4.4 kg of pressure. A "positive" tender point will elicit a dramatic response from your patient ("Ow! Hey, that hurts."). By the fourth tender point, if fibro is present your patient will most definitely not want any more points tested.

Once you are comfortable with your diagnosis, during follow-up visits you need not retest tender points.

The tender points of fibromyalgia

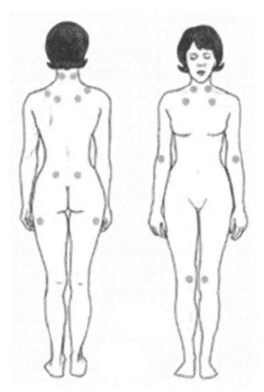

This image has been reproduced with permission from the National Institute of Arthritis and Musculoskeletal and Skin Diseases.

The Fatigue of fibromyalgia

- Unchecked by an adequate serotonin stress-buffering system, the patient's protracted stress triggers non-stop stimulation of her hypothalamic-pituitary-adrenal (HPA) axis. Also affected in the HPA axis are thyroid and ovary.

- Adrenal depletion ("adrenal fatigue"): measurable low DHEA, low cortisol, sluggish response to ACTH stimulation, low norepinephrine. Symptoms: fatigue with afternoon crash, orthostatic hypotension, salt craving.

- Thyroid depletion ("thyroid fatigue"): low TSH, low free T3, low basal body temperature (97.6 or lower). Symptoms: cold hands and feet, dry skin/hair, outer third of eyebrows thinning, weight gain, mental sluggishness.

- Ovarian depletion: low estradiol and progesterone. Symptoms: PMS, lack of libido.

- Other sources of fatigue: inefficient sleep, depression.

- This fatigue is what we all know as Chronic Fatigue Syndrome (CFS), so popular in the 1970s and 1980s as the "yuppie flu." A support group of chronically fatigued patients renamed the condition CFIDS (chronic fatigue immune dysfunction syndrome), although there has never been any research consistently linking chronic fatigue with any infection or any immune dysfunction.

Co-morbidities prevalent with fibromyalgia

- Headaches, tension and migraine (10-80% of fibro patients)

- Major depressive disorder (20-25%)
- Temporomandibular joint disorder (75%)
- Irritable bowel syndrome (30-80%)
- Multiple chemical sensitivities, both environmental and medication triggers (33-55%)
- Chronic pelvic pain, vulvodynia, dyspareunia (20%)

Fibro as a disability

Self-reported by patient herself as "can do with much difficulty" or "unable to perform."

- Heavy household tasks (70% of fibro patients)
- Lifting, carrying 25 lbs without help (60%)
- Strenuous activities (55%)
- Walk one mile (50%)
- Climb one flight of stairs (44%)
- Light household tasks (36%)

The role of a second neurotransmitter, norepinephrine

- Neurotransmitter present in both brain and adrenal gland.
- Plays key role in fight-or-flight response.
- Depleted during protracted adrenal stress in patient with low-serotonin stress susceptibility.
- Low levels associated with depression, apathy, brain fog, increased susceptibility to pain.

Lab tests of fibro patient will demonstrate physiologic changes of protracted stress in a genetically susceptible person (male or female, but usually female). There is *no evidence* of pathology or inflammation with fibro except when a patient has two separate diagnoses (e.g., fibro and rheumatoid arthritis). Physiologic "positive" lab tests:

- Low serotonin.
- Diminished hypothalamic-pituitary-adrenal (HPA) function with adrenal and thyroid "fatigue."
- Sluggish adrenal response to ACTH stimulation.
- Adrenal fatigue: low norepinephrine, low cortisol, low DHEA.
- Thyroid fatigue: low TSH, low or low-normal free T3, T4. Low basal body temperatures (97.6 or lower).

Summary

- Fibro usually begins in a genetically susceptible low-serotonin woman who has endured a period of protracted stress (family stresses, financial stresses, relationship stresses, etc.).

- The women in her family usually have a history of any of the low-serotonin stress susceptibility disorders listed above and/or a history of SSRI use.

- The patient herself may have experienced any of the low-serotonin disorders following stressful episodes in her life. Taking a biographically oriented history will reveal much information in this regard.

- 25% of fibro women experienced emotional, physical, or sexual abuse as children.

- During and after her period of relentless stress, her muscles chronically tightened painfully as if she is trying to defend herself—almost as if she is creating a suit of armor with her muscles.

- Her unchecked fight-or-flight response depletes her thyroid and adrenal glands.

- From chronic pain she becomes depressed, sleeps poorly,

is fatigued, and suffers cognitive difficulties.

- Because her tests are negative, she is written off as depressed and a "whiner." Eventually her symptoms worsen to the extent of rendering her eligible for disability status.

Part 2: When to Suspect Fibromyalgia

If you are a primary care physician, 5 to 7% of your female patients either have fibro or are at significant risk for developing it.

The actual diagnosis of fibro (as described in Part 1) is a clinical one, based on the history you obtain and your physical examination. No lab tests are needed to diagnose fibro. **You do not need to refer any fibro patient to a specialist of any kind.** The American College of Rheumatologists actually discourages fibro referrals. Mayo Clinic no longer accepts fibro or chronic fatigue patients. This one is all yours!

1. **Suspect fibro every time a patient (especially female) says:**

   - "I feel achy all over."

   - "My shoulders and neck feel really tight."

   - "I'm getting these headaches…"

   - "I am so tired all the time."

   - "I have these backaches. I've been seeing a chiropractor, but…"

   - "I just can't seem to get enough sleep. I wake up tired."

   - "I'm depressed."

- "I just don't feel well and I know you told me everything is normal."

Get her up on the table, check her tender points, order basic lab as part of a routine fatigue work-up (blood count, metabolic profile, thyroid profile, sed rate, rheumatoid factor). If she has painful tender points, you have diagnosed fibro

2. **If you have an opportunity to review pertinent biographical data,** ask about family history of depression, anxiety, SSRI use, fibromyalgia, chronic fatigue, migraines, IBS, and other low-serotonin stress susceptibility disorders.

   If you suspect fibro, bring up the childhood abuse issues obliquely, saying something like "With this particular condition, it turns out a lot of the patients had really stressful childhoods, with emotional, physical, and even sexual abuse problems. Looking back on your childhood, would you say yours was a happy one or a stressful one?"

   Women who were abused as children rarely reveal this (especially to a male physician), but they will be grateful to any physician who brings this painful issue into the open. If an abuse issue is present, I myself then say to the patient, "Imagine the posture of a little girl (you) when her abuser comes home." She will likely hunch her shoulders together protectively. I then say, "That's the way your body has learned to deal with stress, tightening your muscles. That is fibromyalgia."

3. **If your patient is being treated for anxiety or depression,** always ask about any chronic physical symptoms, especially muscle pain and fatigue. These

patients seem to never volunteer physical symptoms to their therapists. The therapists rarely ask and virtually never check their client for tender points.

Lab tests to order if you suspect fibro

Beyond the standard fatigue panel mentioned above, I routinely order two lab tests and instruct patient on a self-test, mainly to demonstrate to the patient herself what is happening in her body.

1. **Pharmasan (formerly neuroScience) has developed insurance-reimbursable tests that measure levels of neurotransmitters and adrenal function.** You will dispense a kit to your patient containing a small bottle for urine (second morning specimen) and four small vials for salivary samples throughout a single day.

   Your patient collects the specimens as instructed and mails them directly to the lab.

   - Urine: neurotransmitters>specifically serotonin and norepinephrine.

   - Saliva: cortisol levels throughout a single day and DHEA.

   The results most often confirm what you have inferred: low serotonin and norepinephrine, low DHEA, and low cortisol. (Treatment of any abnormalities follows in Part 3.)

2. **Instructions on self-testing for thyroid fatigue using a basal thermometer.** After five days of taking her basal temperature on waking (use the five days following first day of menstrual flow to avoid the temperature rise of ovulation), if her average is 97.6 or lower, she has mild

hypothyroidism *even with a normal TSH.* Basal temperature testing was a standard means of diagnosing hypothyroidism during the years before the introduction of the TSH measurement in the 1960s. It remains just as useful in this situation in which the pituitary is "fatigued" and unable to produce elevated levels of TSH. (Treatment of any abnormalities follows in Part 3.)

Part 3: Treating Fibro

When treating fibro, it helps to remember how we treat diabetes, another condition affecting millions of Americans. We base our approach to a diabetic depending on the severity of the situation. Mild diabetes really requires only lifestyle changes (weight loss, exercise). Moderate diabetes moves to the oral hypoglycemics. Severe diabetes necessitates adding insulin.

It's pretty much the same with fibro: mild, moderate, severe.

Step 1: Categorize the severity of your patient's fibro.

Mild fibro: Her symptoms have been around one year or less. The stress she knew she carried in her neck and shoulders is now constant and she feels achy over her entire body. She is not disabled, is continuing her usual daily activities, but is aware her symptoms are beginning to interfere with her day-to-day enjoyment of life. She is often too tired after work to consider any evening activities and turns down invitations as "too tired." Although your physical exam will show "positive" tender points, she is startled by their presence. "Wow! That hurts! I didn't know that was there!"

Moderate fibro: Symptoms usually present less than five

years, but are now daily. She awakens stiff, tired, and feeling "old." Your exam reveals painful tender points. She is in pain through the entire day and her daily activities are a struggle. This patient has usually been to several physicians and one may have actually suggested fibro as a diagnosis, but said something like "We don't know much about it" and written her an antidepressant.

Severe fibro: Symptoms longer than five years. Chronic daily severe muscle pain. This patient doesn't even want her skin touched during an exam and a tender point exam will almost invariably bring on sweating and tears. She moves stiffly and slowly and her face is that of a patient in chronic pain. She has often left her job, and is considering or may already be on disability. If married, her husband does most of the housework. Her fibro dominates her life.

Step 2 (applies to all levels of severity): Educate your patient about fibro.

Studies have shown that simple patient education can actually reduce severity of symptoms. Although her fibro was likely triggered by some definable stressor, now years have passed and the stressor is the fibro itself. Once your patient understands that fibro is not a disease, but rather a genetic susceptibility causing her to overreact to stress, she will be less frightened about the possibility of being disabled for the rest of her life. By breaking this stress>pain>increased stress>increased pain cycle, her muscles can start to relax on their own.

Emphasize that because of her unique sensitivity to stress, her muscles have created a suit of armor over her body. Reassure her that fibro does not lead to any disease and that her symptoms can be brought under control. Do caution her that she can't change her genes and she may experience episodic flare-ups of fibro that may necessitate treatment. Common triggers for "fibro-flares" are new stresses in her life, hormonal changes like menopause, physical injury (e.g., a whiplash-inducing auto accident), or even changes in the weather.

Urge your patient to faithfully follow the stress-reduction steps presented in my book, *Healing Fibromyalgia.*

Step 3 (applies to all levels of severity): Consider psychotherapy, especially cognitive behavioral therapy (CBT) if available.

No shortage of studies has confirmed that CBT does help fibro symptoms, teaching your patient to reframe the way she thinks and acts about stressful situations including fibro pain. The major advantage of CBT is that results can begin in as few as four to six sessions and the average number of total sessions is just 16.

Step 4 (applies to all levels of severity): Refer your patient to a physical therapist or chiropractor who is familiar with fibro.

Although exercise will definitely help fibro, most patients respond to the suggestion "Go exercise," by thinking "Who is he kidding?" Remember, fibro patients are tired and depressed and they hurt.

Mild and moderate fibro: Write a physical therapy prescription for a graded exercise program (to recondition her muscles) and authorize six to eight hour-long sessions of specific forms of massage called *myofascial release and deep tissue therapy.* Unlike Swedish massage, which essentially kneads and rubs the muscles, deep tissue work presses into the chronically contracted muscle knots of fibro. Myofascial release stretches the muscles and the tight fascia that is binding them.

Severe fibro: Begin graded exercise only. These patients are simply in too much pain to tolerate myofascial release and deep tissue work. Once symptoms have been controlled with medication, you can prescribe these additional massage therapies.

Step 5 (applies to all levels of severity): My book — *Healing Fibromyalgia* — provides in detail a healthful eating program for fibro.

Please encourage your patient to follow it. Basically, she will replace simple carbohydrates (white flour, sugar) with complex ones, reduce saturated fats, and eliminate junk foods. Sometimes fibro is worsened by gluten, so I encourage all patients to try going one month gluten-free to determine if this may be contributing to symptoms (instructions for the gluten elimination and reintroduction trial are included in the book). Because most fibro patients are overweight, your patient will be encouraged to keep a careful eye on her daily calorie intake.

Step 6: Medications for fibro.

Surveys of physicians who regularly treat fibro have shown that a typical patient with moderate-to-severe symptoms is frequently taking six separate prescriptions a day to keep her symptoms under control. These are commonly:

- One of the FDA-approved fibro medications (Lyrica, Savella, Cymbalta)
- A muscle relaxant (Flexeril, Soma, Skelaxin)

- A sleep med (Ambien, Lunesta)
- A pain med (Vicodin, Tramadol, OxyContin)
- An antidepressant (Lexapro, Effexor)
- An "energizer" (Provigil, Nuvigil)

However, this degree of polypharmacy would only apply to a small number of especially severe fibro patients. Since fibro patients are all chemically sensitive (susceptible to side effects from any or all medications), the best idea is to use as few medications as possible and, for mild cases, rely initially on the lifestyle change therapies described above.

Mild fibro

Because I have had two decades of experience using nutritional supplements in lieu of prescription drugs, I treat mild fibro with the following regimen of five supplements:

- **St. John's wort** 450 mg twice a day (a very mild SSRI).

- **5 Hydroxytryptophan** 100 mg at bedtime (precursor to serotonin, helpful for sleep).

- **D,L Phenylalanine + L Tyrosine** 500 mg daily (many brands available for these amino acids, which are norepinephrine precursors).

Note: Taken together, these three supplements create very mild and side-effect-free versions of Savella and Cymbalta.

- **Theanine** 100 mg three times a day (an amino acid derivative of green tea that acts as mild, nonsedating anxiolytic and muscle relaxant).

- **Magnesium/malic acid** (many brands): A popular over-the-counter combination for fibro. Magnesium acting as a muscle relaxant, malic acid (the same one from Krebs Citric Acid cycle) to improve energy and sense of well-being.

AND

1. **If basal temperatures average 97.6 or lower,** start Armour thyroid ½ gr. (30 mg.) or Synthroid 50 mcg each morning. This is basically a physiologic dose of replacement hormone and can be discontinued in 6 to 9 months. This small dose will not induce hyperthyroid symptoms or pose any risks.

2. **Based on cortisol and DHEA levels from Pharmasan Labs,** if cortisol levels are low, start Cortef 10 mg in AM, 5 mg in afternoon and/or DHEA 10 mg each morning.

Note: This is basically a physiologic replacement dose of cortisone and has minimal anti-inflammatory effect. I generally continue this after about three months of good pain control (the chronic pain itself being responsible for adrenal "fatigue"). Once her pain has been controlled and her stress reduced, her adrenal function will normalize on its own. Remember there is no adrenal "disease" (like Addison's disease) only "fatigue."

Moderate fibro

Generally, the mild nutritional supplements used for mild fibro will not be sufficient to control symptoms of moderately severe fibro (although many patients, remembering side effects they've experienced in the past, may prefer to try nutritional supplement therapy for several weeks). When switching from supplements to medications, I discontinue the St. John's wort, 5HTP, and the D,L Phenylalanine/Tyrosine. Unlike prescription SSRIs or SNRIs, these supplements do not need to be tapered. Drug recommendations for moderate fibro follow directly.

FDA-approved fibro drugs: Savella and Cymbalta

Although completely different molecules, Savella and Cymbalta work alike, by raising both serotonin and norepinephrine (DNRI=dual neurotransmitter reuptake inhibitors). I am uncertain why both manufacturers state something along the lines of "we don't know how these work."

Raising serotonin will raise your patient's stress buffer, just like any SSRI. Raising norepinephrine restores levels to her depleted adrenal, increases energy, and improves pain control. That's how they work.

Having used both medications in hundreds of fibro patients, let me warn you against the package insert of FDA-approved dosing instructions. With both Savella and Cymbalta, the recommended starting doses for both are too high and ramp-up to maintenance too quick for most fibromyalgia patients to tolerate. Following the guidelines will usually result in side effects of sufficient severity for your patient to abandon her medication. If the drugs are taken as per the insert, your patient's norepinephrine will rise too quickly and she'll feel extremely nauseated. The key to these medicines: *go slowly!*

Savella

Instead of Forest Labs recommendation to reach maintenance (50 mg BID) in seven days, **allow six weeks to reach this dose.** At this rate, she will feel maximum benefit at eight weeks.

I write three separate prescriptions for Savella, cleverly numbering them #1, #2, and #3:

Prescription #1 Savella 12.5 mg Disp. 60. One tab qhs x 5 nights, followed by one tab BID x 7 days, followed by one tab in AM, two tabs qhs x 7 days, followed by two tabs BID until supply is used up.

Then fill Prescription #2 Savella 25 mg Disp 60. One tab BID x 7 days, then one tab qAM and 2 tabs qhs X 14 days, then two tabs BID until supply used up.

Lastly fill Prescription #3 Savella 50 mg BID (maintenance).

Notes

- If severe nausea develops with any dose increase, return to the previously tolerated dose and remain there for two weeks before attempting to increase it again.

- If good relief occurs at a lower dose than 50 mg BID, simply remain there.

- If Savella fails to offer good relief, consider adding a small dose of Lyrica (see below) or even OxyContin (10-20 mg q 12 hr).

Cymbalta

The same gradual increase as Savella is necessary:

Prescription #1 Cymbalta 20 mg Disp 30 (maximum allowed by insurance)
Prescription #2 Cymbalta 30 mg Disp 30
Prescription #3 Cymbalta 60 mg Disp 30

Note

- Make sure your patient fills these on different days or they will all be denied by her insurer.

Week one: Cymbalta 20 mg qAM

Week two: Cymbalta 30 mg qAM
Week three: Cymbalta 40 mg qAM (two 20s)
Week four: Cymbalta 50 mg qAM (one 20 mg and one 30 mg)
Week five: Cymbalta 60 mg qAM (maintenance)

Notes

- If severe nausea develops with any dose increase, return to the previously tolerated dose and remain there for two weeks before attempting to increase it again.

- If good relief occurs at a lower dose than 50 mg BID, simply remain there.

- If Cymbalta fails to offer good relief, consider adding a small dose of Lyrica (see below) or even OxyContin (10-20 mg q 12 hr).

Lyrica

This is a medication for all neuropathic pain, originally approved for diabetic and herpetic neuropathy. For fibro patients, it works by reducing the release of pain modulating neurotransmitters (glutamate and Substance P).

Side effects can be troubling and include dizziness, nausea, brain fog, ataxia, and weight gain. This last is especially problematic as most fibro patients are already overweight. They must be warned about this side effect and advised to watch their weight carefully, reducing calories if needed. (I cannot guarantee your personal safety when your patient learns that the 25 lbs she added in a year is from the med you prescribed.)

Like the other fibro medications, package insert directions ramp the dose up too quickly.

Lyrica comes in many capsule sizes: 25 mg, 50 mg, 75 mg, 100 mg, 150 mg.

Prescription #1 Lyrica 25 mg Disp 60
Prescription #2 Lyrica 50 mg Disp 60
Prescription #3 Lyrica 75 mg Disp 60
Prescription #4 Lyrica 150 mg Disp 60 (maintenance)

Again, remind the patient not to fill all prescriptions on the same day or they will be denied by her insurer.

Start at 25 mg at bedtime and increase by 25 mg weekly until you reach maintenance at 150 mg BID. A smaller maintenance dose will suffice if this is being used in combination with Savella or Cymbalta.

A USEFUL TIP: A very effective and well-tolerated medication schedule is to combine Savella or Cymbalta with Lyrica, using half doses of each. This actually makes good pharmacologic sense: Savella/Cymbalta raise serotonin/norepinephrine, while Lyrica blocks release of pain modulators. Since these may take several weeks to show clinical benefit, I also prescribe Tramadol ER, 100-200 mg each morning, to give my patient more immediate pain relief.

Notes

- If severe nausea develops with any dose increase, return to the previously tolerated dose and remain there for two weeks before attempting to increase it again.

- If good relief occurs at a lower dose than 50 mg BID, simply remain there.

- If Savella fails to offer good relief, consider adding a small dose of OxyContin (10-20 mg q 12 hr).

For patients with moderate fibro, I add:

Flexeril (cyclobenzaprine) 10 mg OR Trazodone 50 mg at bedtime to deepen sleep and relax muscles.

AND

Tramadol ER 100-200 mg in the morning for all-day pain relief. As the Savella/Cymbalta/Lyrica take effect, this can be discontinued. When you prescribe Tramadol with Savella or Cymbalta, you will invariably receive a telephone call from the pharmacist concerned about serotonin syndrome issues. I have never seen this and when I attended a fibro meeting in New York, none of the 250 physician attendees had ever seen it either.

If the Tramadol is ineffective, I will allow the patient Vicodin 5-10/500 up to TID or OxyContin 10-20 mg q 12 hr. Again, these can be lowered or even discontinued in the future.

For patients with severe fibro:

These patients are virtually incapacitated by their chronic pain and pervasive exhaustion. They are depressed and frustrated by their steady functional decline. Interestingly, though you'll not see many men with fibro, when you do encounter them their fibro is usually in this "severe" category, because they usually have postponed for years (and sometimes decades) seeing anyone for help.

These patients are not difficult to manage provided you are willing to prescribe opioids for the non-cancer pain of fibro. Because fibro patients are extremely sensitive to medications, relatively small doses of opioids can have dramatic beneficial effects. You are using them to break the pain>stress>more pain>more stress cycle while simultaneously adjusting serotonin, norepinephrine, and the pain-modulating neurotransmitters (glutamate and substance P) with Savella, Cymbalta, and/or Lyrica.

Even in the best cases, published studies on these three FDA-approved fibro meds show efficacy rate of only 45%. That means 55% of fibro patients taking these meds do not attain good relief. If Savella/Cymbalta aren't working, add Lyrica, or vice versa, but don't give up. Adding opioids here can really help.

If, for whatever reason, you feel reluctant prescribing opioids for severe fibro pain, then refer your patient to a pain specialist. Please do not allow your patient to spend her life in pain because of a personal bias against these highly effective medications.

Therefore, for severe fibro patients, follow all the steps described for moderate fibro (including Savella/Cymbalta and/or Lyrica and the Flexeril) except instead of Tramadol ER, prescribe:

OxyContin 10 mg every 12 hours and give your patient permission to increase her dose to 20 mg every 12 hours after a week if she is not feeling improvement. You can also allow her up to three (no more) Vicodin 5/500 per day for breakthrough pain.

Re-evaluate her status in about two weeks (if she is taking 2 to 10 mg OxyContin tablets twice a day, she will be running out of medication). This particular dose (i.e., OxyContin 20 mg q 12 hr, with up to three Vicodin 5/500 per day for breakthrough pain) works nicely for the majority of my severe fibro patients.

Approximately 10% require 30 mg q 12 hr and 5% 40 mg q 12 hr. I never go beyond 40 mg every 12 hours. No matter how severe a patient's fibro pain may be, that particular dose—40 mg q 12 hr—is the limit. Virtually no one wants more and were they to ask for more I say, "After 1,600 fibro patients, I known pretty much how much OxyContin is needed. More is not better." Instead, I would prescribe additional physical therapy, myofascial release, and increase Savella, Cymbalta, or Lyrica, but I never increase the opioids beyond this dose.

If, after several months, the OxyContin appears to be less effective, using an online dose comparison chart you can switch to Opana ER, Avinza, Fentanyl patches, or Kadian. The goal, however, is to start lowering doses after several pain-free or at least pain-reduced months. I generally reduce OxyContin by 5 to 10 mg per week. If patients have been following all the lifestyle suggestions, physical therapy exercises, stress reduction techniques, etc, most severe fibro patients can be tapered off their OxyContin in a year and off their FDA-approved meds in 1 ½ to 2 years. They are cautioned about the possibility of "fibro flares" but not to lose heart as these flares are almost always temporary events.

Other medications to consider for moderate and severe fibro

Amrix 15 mg is an extended-release form of cyclobenzaprine (Flexeril) and currently undergoing clinical trials for fibro. In my own experience, I find this an excellent choice and am sure it will get its FDA approval. Using Amrix has allowed to me to avoid opioids or keep the opioid dose low. However, Amrix is very expensive and many insurers balk at paying for Amrix as maintenance therapy.

Xyrem (sodium exacerbate) Clinical trials on what is a reconfiguration of the date-rape drug from the 1970s (gamma hydroxybutyrate) actually showed efficacy in relieving fibro pain by increasing depth of sleep. However, despite good data the FDA quite reasonably turned down the application, fearing widespread abuse potential. In my own experience, Xyrem is effective for those patients who report fibro prevents them "from ever sleeping deeply" and when the regular hypnotics (Ambien, Lunesta, etc.) don't work.

N.B. A recent price increase by Jazz Pharmaceuticals, makers of Xyrem, has pretty much eliminated it from my fibro armamentarium. $4,200 a month. Need I say more?

Butrans (buprenorphine) This is an opioid derivative absorbed through skin and administered as a skin patch once weekly. Sizes are 5, 10, and 20 mcg per hour. The patients I have started on Butrans uniformly reported "no relief" at 5 mcg/hour and "very good" pain relief at 10 mcg/hour. I have not needed to increase it beyond that dose.

Provigil, Nuvigil These are FDA-approved for chronic daytime sleepiness and shift worker sleep disorder. These medications are frequently prescribed off-label for chronic fatigue syndrome, which is essentially the fatigue component of fibro. Patients take this on arising (usually ½ tablet of the lowest dose will suffice) and report sufficient energy and mental clarity to continue through a workday.

Conclusion

To me, one of the most interesting questions to ask ourselves about fibro concerns the status of women in our society. If fibro is essentially an unchecked stress response and 96% of fibro patients are female, have we really made life so stressful for half the occupants of our planet that they need antidepressants and opioids simply to survive?

When we prescribe a serotonin-boosting *anything*—whether it's for anxiety, depression, or fibro—we are essentially raising a person's stress-buffering system. But women given antidepressants report feeling "numb" and "like zombies." Artists on antidepressants report losing their creative spark.

It well may be that the low serotonin level in women (and probably artists as well) places the human stress buffer where it actually should be. After all, women are more intuitive and more sensitive to color, texture, and sensation. They are compassionate in a way that men simply are not.

We need to consider what fibro is trying to say to us about the status of women on our planet, and about the real status of ourselves.

ABOUT THE AUTHORS

David Edelberg, MD, a practicing physician for 30 years, has treated more than 1,600 women with fibromyalgia.

Board-certified in Internal Medicine in 1974, he began incorporating alternative therapies into his practice during the 1980s. Since founding the parent company of WholeHealth Chicago in 1993, he has become nationally recognized as a pioneer in integrative medicine, a specialty combining conventional medicine with alternative therapies.

As senior staff clinician at WholeHealth Chicago Lincoln Park, on Chicago's north side, Dr Edelberg cares for patients with a focus on wellness, disease prevention, and slowing down the inevitable process of getting older.

His free weekly Health Tips offer thought-provoking commentary on medicine and health and are widely praised by his thousands of loyal readers. Register to receive them at wholehealthchicago.com.

Dr. Edelberg has written extensively on complementary and alternative medicine in books for the general public and also for physicians considering career changes to integrative medicine. He teaches alternative and integrative medicine to medical students and residents at the University of Illinois and the University of Chicago, usually providing their first exposure to alternative medicine. He is also assistant professor of medicine at Rush Medical College.

His book, *The Triple Whammy Cure: The Breakthrough Women's Health Program for Feeling Good Again in 3 Weeks*, was published by Free Press in 2006.

Dr. Edelberg is on the Rodale Medical Advisory Board, has served on the board of the American Holistic Medicine Association, and is president of the board of Facets Multimedia, a not-for-profit center of art and foreign film in Chicago, where he lives with his wife and two sons.

"One morning recently, it came to me that on virtually every working day for the past 30 years I've been taking care of patients one-on-one, listening as people revealed their lives and pains, their anxieties and worst fears. It also occurred to me that I'm lucky to still immensely enjoy what I do and that I was actually looking forward to the patients I'd be seeing later that afternoon because I truly feel I'm helping them. Looking back over those three decades, I decided the five finest words any doctor can ever hear are: I think I'm feeling better."

Heidi Hough has collaborated for more than 25 years with physicians, publishers, and websites to develop health and wellness information. She partnered with Dr Edelberg on *The Triple Whammy Cure* and continues to collaborate with him on his weekly health tips.

In 2010, she worked with Arizona-based Brainstorms to write, edit, and shape content for the My Healing Kitchen website, focusing on food and its relationship to wellness and disease, as well as writing and editing *The 30-Day Diabetes Cure*.

Ms Hough and her colleagues teamed with Simon &

Schuster and physicians at Harvard Medical School to conceive, write, and edit the *Harvard Medical School Family Health Guide*, a million-word illustrated consumer health reference. Amazon.com named the book one of the ten best consumer medical books of 1999.

Ms Hough spent 12 years as Editorial Director of the American Medical Association (AMA) Consumer Publishing Division, where she directed the development of 30 consumer books, including the bestselling *AMA Family Medical Guide*, the James Beard Award-winning *AMA Family Cookbook*, the *AMA Encyclopedia of Medicine*, and the 19-volume *AMA Home Medical Library*.

Made in the USA
Lexington, KY
27 January 2019